FUN THINGS TO DO IN RETIREMENT

365 Daily Discoveries of Exciting Adventures and Healthy Pursuits for the Young-at-Heart Seniors

Serena Mitchell

Copyright © 2023 Serena Mitchell

All rights reserved

The characters and events portrayed in this book are fictitious. Any similarity to real persons, living or dead, is coincidental and not intended by the author.

No part of this book may be reproduced, or stored in a retrieval system, or transmitted in any form or by any means, electronic, mechanical, photocopying, recording, or otherwise, without express written permission of the publisher.
The content of this book is provided for purely informational purposes and does not claim to replace professional, medical, legal, or any other type of advice. Although the author and publisher have made every effort to ensure that the information contained in this book is accurate and reflects current thinking at the time of publication, they cannot be held liable for any errors, omissions, or outcomes resulting from using this information. Neither the author nor the publisher will be responsible for any direct or indirect damages that may arise in connection with the use or failure to apply the information and advice proposed in this book. Readers are encouraged to consult competent professionals before making any decision based on the content of this book. The purchase and use of this book imply the reader's acceptance of this disclaimer.

Cover design by: Serena Mitchell
Independently published
ISBN-13: 9798854596701
Printed in the United States of America

CONTENTS

Title Page

Copyright

Introduction

Chapter 1: Embark on Your Adventure - Unleash the Thrill of   1
Retirement Exploration!

Chapter 2. Nature Adventures   8

Chapter 3: Creative and Artistic Pursuits   27

Chapter 4: Fitness and Wellness   34

Chapter 5: Travel and Global Adventures   41

Chapter 6: Cooking and Gastronomy   50

Chapter 7: DIY Projects and Crafts   59

Chapter 8: Cultural Experiences   68

Chapter 9: Socialization and Community   76

Chapter 10: Mindful Wellness and Meditation   84

Chapter 11: Technology and Digital Adventures   93

INTRODUCTION

Welcome to the next chapter of your life, where the journey of retirement unfolds with boundless opportunities for joy, discovery, and fulfillment. Retirement is not merely a destination but a transformative phase that beckons you to embrace new adventures, passions, and experiences like never before. In this exciting new book, "Fun Things to Do in Retirement: 365 Daily Discoveries of Exciting Adventures and Healthy Pursuits for the Young-at-Heart Seniors", we invite you to embark on an extraordinary expedition through a year filled with exhilarating activities, creative pursuits, and a renewed zest for life.

A New Chapter Awaits

As you bid farewell to the daily grind of work, a fresh chapter opens before you – one filled with unexplored avenues and infinite possibilities. Retirement is not about stepping back; it's about stepping forward into a realm of endless freedom where your desires, passions, and dreams take center stage. Whether you've been looking forward to this phase for years or the concept of retirement is a recent revelation, we assure you that this is a journey that will redefine the meaning of retirement entirely.

Unlocking the Treasure Trove of Adventure

In "Fun Things to Do in Retirement," we've curated a treasure trove of activities that will light up your days and enrich your life. Each day brings a delightful surprise – a carefully selected adventure or pursuit to ignite your curiosity and stimulate your senses. From invigorating outdoor escapades to stimulating intellectual explorations, there's something to captivate every soul. Whether you're a seasoned retiree seeking to revitalize your daily routine or someone newly entering the world of retirement with a zeal for exploration, this book is tailor-made to make every day a celebration of living life to the fullest.

The Essence of Adventurous Living

In retirement, life becomes a blank canvas awaiting your creative brushstrokes. Our book celebrates the essence of adventurous living, where curiosity thrives, and boredom finds no place. Engage in nature's wonders with awe-inspiring hikes, indulge in artistic pursuits that nourish the soul, and embark on culinary journeys that delight the taste buds. For the spirited traveler, there are virtual expeditions to far-off lands and opportunities to volunteer and make a meaningful impact across the globe.

Cultivating Holistic Well-being

Retirement is the ideal time to prioritize your well-being, nurturing both mind and body. We understand the significance of holistic health and have curated activities that focus on mindfulness, meditation, and gentle exercises to promote tranquility and balance. Engage in the ancient arts of Tai Chi and Qi Gong to awaken your energy or participate in wellness retreats that rejuvenate the spirit.

Embracing the Digital Age

In a world driven by technology, we recognize the importance of staying connected and utilizing digital resources for continued growth. Our book ventures into the realm of digital adventures, where virtual travel experiences and online learning open doors to unparalleled opportunities. Embrace your creative side with digital art and storytelling, showcasing that age knows no bounds when it comes to technological empowerment.

A Roadmap for Endless Inspiration

"Fun Things to Do in Retirement: 365 Daily Discoveries of Exciting Adventures and Healthy Pursuits for the Young-at-Heart Seniors" is not just a book; it's your roadmap to endless inspiration and self-discovery. We've thoughtfully crafted each activity to cater to the desires of young-at-heart seniors like you. Whether you're seeking camaraderie with like-minded individuals through book clubs and hobby groups or eager to pass on your wisdom through mentorship and volunteering, there's an enriching experience for everyone.

Your Invitation to Adventure

The world is brimming with wonders awaiting your exploration. Embrace the spirit of adventure and awaken the joy that resides within. Each page of this book is an invitation to discover the wonders that retirement has to offer. Let your heart soar with excitement as you turn each page, anticipating the magic of a new adventure.

"Fun Things to Do in Retirement: 365 Daily Discoveries of Exciting Adventures and Healthy Pursuits for the Young-at-Heart Seniors" is your companion on this incredible journey of discovery and celebration. As you immerse yourself in these activities, remember that retirement is not the end of a chapter but the beginning of an enthralling new narrative. So, dear reader, are you ready to seize the reins of this thrilling adventure? Embark on the journey of a lifetime, and let the exploration begin!

CHAPTER 1: EMBARK ON YOUR ADVENTURE - UNLEASH THE THRILL OF RETIREMENT EXPLORATION!

Retirement is not the end; it's the beginning of an exhilarating journey filled with endless possibilities! In "Fun Things to Do in Retirement: 365 Daily Discoveries of Exciting Adventures and Healthy Pursuits for the Young-at-Heart Seniors", we invite you to embark on an adventure that will ignite your passion for exploration and discovery like never before.

Discover New Horizons

Retirement offers the remarkable opportunity to break free from the confines of routine and step boldly into uncharted territories. As the curtains rise on this new phase of life, you'll find yourself standing at the threshold of endless adventures, waiting to be embraced. Shed the weight of daily obligations and let your spirit soar with newfound freedom. Embrace the thrill of exploration as you dive headfirst into activities that once lingered on the periphery of your busy life.

Retirement isn't a time to settle; it's an invitation to seek out new horizons and expand your horizons. You may uncover a hidden talent for painting, capturing the beauty of life with every stroke of the brush. Or perhaps you'll discover a passion for hiking, immersing yourself in the breathtaking vistas of nature's grandeur. With each day, a world of possibilities unfolds, offering you the chance to indulge in pursuits that bring joy and fulfillment to your soul.

Gone are the days of adhering to rigid schedules; this is the time to embrace spontaneity and curiosity. It's time to say "yes" to experiences you've always yearned for but never had the chance to explore. Whether it's signing up for that art class you've been eyeing, learning a new language to connect with different cultures, or embarking on a solo road trip to soak in the beauty of distant landscapes, the canvas of retirement awaits your vibrant brushstrokes.

The path ahead may be uncharted, but it's precisely this sense of novelty that makes the journey exhilarating. Embrace each new day as an opportunity to venture into the unknown, knowing that every step will lead you closer to discovering the depths of your passions and the vastness of your potential. Retirement is an invitation to bloom anew, to set aside preconceived notions, and to relish in the thrill of the unexpected.

So, dear reader, as you embark on this exhilarating adventure of retirement exploration, remember that the horizon stretches far beyond what you can see. Discover the joys of a life unbounded by limitations and relish in the thrill of discovering new facets of yourself. Let "Fun Things to Do in Retirement" be your compass, guiding you toward an extraordinary journey of self-discovery, wonder, and excitement. The thrill of retirement exploration awaits; embrace it with open arms and an adventurous spirit!

A Year of Adventure Awaits

Picture this: 365 days filled with boundless excitement and endless possibilities. Each morning, you wake up with a sense of anticipation, knowing that the day ahead holds a thrilling adventure crafted just for you. In "Fun Things to Do in Retirement," we've meticulously curated a year-long calendar of exhilarating activities, ensuring that your journey into retirement is nothing short of extraordinary.

From the first rays of dawn to the enchanting dusk, we have something special in store for every day of the year. Each activity is a gateway to new experiences, inviting you to savor the richness of life from various angles. The thoughtfully crafted itinerary includes an array of adventures, catering to the diverse interests and passions that make you who you are. For the nature enthusiast, we have awe-inspiring hikes that lead you through lush forests and breathtaking landscapes. Wander through the beauty of the great outdoors and reconnect with Mother Nature in her purest form. Allow the whispering winds and rustling leaves to be your guide, as you embark on a soul-nourishing journey amidst the wonders of the natural world.

Are you an artistic soul seeking creative expression? Delve into the realms of art and culture as we present an array of artistic pursuits to ignite your imagination. Engage your senses with painting, writing, and crafting – each stroke of the brush and every word on the page is an opportunity to express the essence of your being.

For the gourmands and culinary enthusiasts, prepare to tantalize your taste buds with a delectable array of gastronomic delights. Embark on a culinary journey that transcends borders, as we explore diverse cuisines from around the world. Delight in the aroma of freshly baked bread and let the spices of far-off lands transport you to distant shores.

As the seasons change, so do the activities. From cozy winter retreats to blossoming spring escapades, each chapter of the year brings with it unique experiences and cherished memories. Allow the turning of the calendar to be a testament to the richness of life, where every day is an opportunity to create lasting moments.

So, whether you choose to embark on this adventure solo or share the experience with loved ones, know that "365 Fun Things to Do in Retirement" is your compass. It will guide you through a year that promises to be filled with laughter, learning, and boundless joy.

As the pages of this book unfurl, your year of adventure awaits, and with it, a profound transformation of your perspective on retirement. Embrace this unique opportunity to awaken the adventurer within and let the enchantment of each day lead you toward a life of wonder and fulfillment. Together, let's make this year in retirement a celebration of living fully and unapologetically, where each sunrise is a new chance to explore, and each sunset is a moment of gratitude for a life well-lived. Welcome to your year of extraordinary adventures – are you ready to seize the day?

Fuel Your Wanderlust

Within the boundless realm of retirement, the allure of exploration beckons with an irresistible charm. Prepare to awaken your inner wanderer as we delve into a world of travel and adventure, designed to ignite your wanderlust and spark a sense of wonder for the unknown.

In "Fun Things to Do in Retirement: 365 Daily Discoveries of Exciting Adventures and Healthy Pursuits for the Young-at-Heart Seniors", we recognize that travel is not just about ticking destinations off a bucket list; it's a transformative journey that enriches the soul. Whether you dream of traversing distant lands or savoring the beauty of your own backyard, we have an array of travel experiences to satisfy your longing for discovery.

Explore the breathtaking landscapes of far-off lands through the captivating lens of virtual travel experiences. From the ancient wonders of historical cities to the serene shores of tropical paradises, you'll find yourself immersed in a kaleidoscope of cultures and traditions, all from the comfort of your own home.

For those yearning for a more tangible escapade, embrace the spirit of road trips – an iconic symbol of freedom and adventure. Hit the open road with a sense of spontaneity and allow the winding highways to lead you to new destinations and hidden gems. Witness the changing scenery as you journey through picturesque landscapes, uncovering the beauty that lies beyond the horizon.

Beyond the allure of distant shores, we invite you to embrace the concept of "slow travel." Delve into the heart of local communities, and forge connections that transcend cultural boundaries. Engage in cultural exchanges, participate in traditional rituals, and savor authentic flavors that capture the essence of each destination. Whether it's strolling through vibrant markets, joining local celebrations, or simply engaging in heartfelt conversations with the locals, slow travel allows you to immerse yourself fully in the tapestry of a new place.

If wanderlust calls you to serve beyond borders, embark on travel volunteering opportunities that make a meaningful impact on communities around the world. Share your skills, expertise, and compassionate heart with those in need, and experience the profound joy that comes from making a difference in the lives of others. Travel with purpose and leave behind a trail of kindness and hope, making the world a better place, one small act of kindness at a time.

From virtual voyages to in-person escapades, "Fun Things to Do in Retirement" encapsulates the essence of travel as a transformative force that expands our horizons and fosters a sense of global interconnectedness. Our goal is to ignite your passion for exploration and inspire you to embrace travel as a catalyst for personal growth and enlightenment.

So, whether you're setting foot on foreign soil or voyaging through the digital realm, let "Fun Things to Do in Retirement: 365 Daily Discoveries of Exciting Adventures and Healthy Pursuits for the Young-at-Heart Seniors" be your compass to navigate the vast seas of wanderlust. Fuel your sense of adventure and let the thrill of travel shape your retirement journey into a tale of wander, discovery, and boundless joy. The world awaits – are you ready to answer the call of wanderlust?

CHAPTER 2. NATURE ADVENTURES

Scenic Hikes: Spectacular Routes and Breathtaking Trails to Explore

If you love immersing yourself in the pristine beauty of nature, breathtaking landscapes, and the refreshing air of hiking trails, then this chapter will guide you to discover thrilling hikes. The "Scenic Hikes" offer an engaging and rejuvenating experience, allowing you to connect with the magnificence of nature during your retirement journey.

This chapter will take you through a selection of spectacular routes and trails that will leave you in awe. You'll have the opportunity to explore majestic mountain ranges, traverse enchanting forests, stroll along stunning coastal vistas, and reach panoramic summits offering unparalleled views.

Each route will be accompanied by a detailed description of the surrounding environment's features and unique characteristics, along with helpful tips for preparing for the hike. You'll also find information about the trail's difficulty level and recommended gear to ensure a smooth and enjoyable experience.

From the more accessible paths to the more challenging ones,

"Scenic Hikes" is designed to satisfy the adventurous appetite of every hiker, allowing you to fully immerse yourself in nature and discover remote corners of unspoiled beauty. Whether you're an experienced hiker or a curious beginner, this chapter will inspire you to embark on thrilling journeys filled with natural discoveries and moments of serene reflection.

Pack your backpacks, lace up your comfortable shoes, and get ready to explore postcard-perfect vistas and create unforgettable memories during your retirement's "Scenic Hikes." Nature awaits you with open arms, ready to unveil its beauty with every step of the way.

A Symphony of Nature's Beauty

As you embark on your "Scenic Hikes," be prepared to immerse yourself in a symphony of nature's beauty. Each trail you tread will lead you through a mesmerizing overture of sights and sounds, captivating your senses and stirring your soul.

The majestic mountain ranges will stand tall like grand symphony conductors, orchestrating the breathtaking panorama that unfolds before your eyes. Towering peaks will reach for the sky, while lush valleys will lay out a verdant carpet at your feet. The soft murmur of a nearby stream will add a delicate note to the symphony, providing a soothing backdrop to your journey.

As you traverse through enchanting forests, the rustling leaves and gentle whispers of the trees will serenade you, creating a harmonious melody with every step you take. Sunlight filtering through the foliage will cast dancing shadows, like musical notes on a sheet, guiding your path with a natural rhythm.

The coastal vistas will add a touch of grandeur to the symphony, with the crashing waves composing a powerful percussion section. Seabirds will join in with their cheerful calls, adding a lively cadence to the symphony of the sea.

When you ascend to panoramic summits, the symphony will crescendo to its peak, offering you a triumphant finale of awe-inspiring views. The vast expanse of the landscape below will stretch like a symphonic score, telling the story of nature's timeless beauty.

As you listen to this symphony of nature's beauty, take a moment to be present in the orchestra of life. Let the sights and sounds seep into your being, filling your heart with gratitude and wonder. Each hike will offer you a unique movement, a chance to experience the symphony from a different vantage point, leaving you with memories that resonate like musical notes in your soul.

In the grand symphony of life, these "Scenic Hikes" will be some of the most memorable movements. They will remind you that retirement is not merely a period of rest but an opportunity to be part of the eternal symphony of nature's wonders. So, let the music guide your steps, and may you find harmony and joy in every note along the way.

The Call of the Mountains

Among the diverse "Scenic Hikes" that await you, none are as captivating as those that answer the call of the mountains. These majestic peaks beckon adventurers with their awe-inspiring allure and hold the promise of unparalleled vistas and a profound sense of accomplishment.

As you ascend the rugged trails, you will feel an irresistible pull, drawing you closer to the summit. The mountains stand as timeless sentinels, whispering tales of resilience and strength to those who dare to conquer their heights. Each step is a testament to your determination and a celebration of the human spirit's indomitable nature.

The ascent is not merely a physical endeavor; it becomes a spiritual journey, too. Surrounded by the untouched beauty of nature, you will find solace and a profound connection to the earth beneath your feet. The mountains' embrace will fill you with a sense of humility, as you witness the grandeur of the world from their lofty perch.

As you ascend, the air grows crisper, and the world below shrinks to a mere glimpse. Time seems to stand still, and you become part of a larger symphony that harmonizes with the elements. With each step, you leave behind the mundane and ascend towards a higher perspective, both literally and figuratively.

Upon reaching the summit, a breathtaking panorama unfolds before your eyes. The mountains' call has led you to a place of rare beauty and tranquility. As you stand at the peak, the world below seems to pause, and you become one with the mountains themselves.

The mountains whisper to your soul, inviting you to embrace the profound serenity they offer. In their presence, worries dissipate, and clarity takes hold. The experience of conquering a mountain is a reminder that challenges are meant to be overcome, and with determination, one can surmount any obstacle.

The descent brings its own sense of fulfillment and gratitude. As you retrace your steps, you carry the memory of the mountains within you, knowing that their call will forever resonate in your heart.

So, heed the call of the mountains as you embark on your "Scenic Hikes." Let their majestic allure guide your journey and leave you with a renewed appreciation for the beauty of nature and the strength within yourself. The mountains await your ascent, ready to bestow their wisdom and beauty upon those who dare to listen to their call.

Lush Forests and Enchanted Woodlands

Step into a world of wonder as you venture into the realm of lush forests and enchanted woodlands during your "Scenic Hikes." Nature's emerald havens await, inviting you to immerse yourself in the serenity and enchantment they offer.

As you enter the embrace of the forest, a symphony of life surrounds you. The rustling leaves whisper secrets of ages past, and the gentle sway of branches creates a soothing melody. Sunlight filters through the canopy, casting dappled patterns on the forest floor, leading you further into the heart of this magical realm.

Every step through the undergrowth reveals hidden treasures. Discover delicate wildflowers painting the forest floor with their vibrant hues and encounter ancient trees that have stood witness to countless seasons. The air is imbued with the earthy fragrance of moss and fallen leaves, creating a scent that evokes a sense of grounding and peace.

Enchanted woodlands unveil hidden nooks and mysterious clearings, as if nature herself has woven a tapestry of secrets for you to explore. As you walk deeper into the forest's embrace, time seems to slow, and the outside world fades away. Here, in the tranquility of nature, you find respite from the hustle and bustle of everyday life.

Birdsong fills the air, and if you listen closely, you may catch a glimpse of elusive woodland creatures gracefully moving through the foliage. Every corner holds the promise of new discoveries, inviting you to be present and embrace the magic of the moment.

The forest's enchantment extends beyond sight and sound; it touches something deeper within. It evokes a sense of wonder, igniting the imagination and rekindling a childlike curiosity for the mysteries of the natural world.

As you traverse the winding trails, you'll feel a profound connection with the forest and the life it sustains. It becomes a sanctuary, a place to find solace, and a source of inspiration that nourishes the soul.

Lush forests and enchanted woodlands offer more than a hike; they grant you entry into a realm of enchantment, where the ordinary becomes extraordinary, and the mundane transforms into magic. So, let the allure of these verdant realms guide your footsteps, and allow yourself to be enchanted by the timeless beauty and grace of the forest.

Cascading Waterfalls and Serene Streams

Within the enchanting world of "Scenic Hikes," you'll encounter the mesmerizing allure of cascading waterfalls and serene streams. These natural wonders offer a symphony of sights and sounds, beckoning you to experience the soothing embrace of flowing water.

As you approach a cascading waterfall, the sound of rushing water grows louder, like nature's own melody. The sight of water tumbling over rocky ledges creates a captivating display of raw power and beauty. The mist that rises from the waterfall kisses your skin, leaving you feeling refreshed and invigorated.

Each waterfall has its unique personality, some roaring with thunderous force, while others gracefully cascade in gentle tiers. Capturing the perfect photograph of these marvels becomes a delightful challenge as you attempt to freeze a moment of their eternal dance.

Following the trail along serene streams is a journey of tranquility. The gentle babbling of water over pebbles creates a serene ambiance, inviting you to relax and let go of any lingering worries. The crystal-clear waters mirror the surrounding foliage, forming a tranquil painting that showcases nature's artistry.

As you walk alongside these peaceful streams, you'll discover hidden nooks and secluded spots perfect for moments of quiet reflection. The rhythmic flow of the water seems to echo the pace of your own thoughts, soothing the mind and calming the soul.

Whether you choose to stand in awe before a majestic waterfall or walk along a serene stream, these water features hold a magical power over the human spirit. They inspire a sense of awe for the grandeur of nature and remind us of the cyclical flow of life.

Cascading waterfalls and serene streams offer a visual and auditory feast, inviting you to reconnect with the beauty of the natural world. Allow yourself to be captivated by the symphony of water's movement, and let the gentle melodies wash away any stresses, leaving you with a sense of peace and wonder. In these moments, you'll find a deeper connection with the rhythmic heartbeat of nature, leaving you with cherished memories to carry in your heart long after the hike is over.

Preserving Nature's Treasures

As you embark on your "Scenic Hikes" through the awe-inspiring landscapes, you'll find yourself surrounded by nature's precious treasures. In this subsection, we explore the importance of preserving these natural wonders for future generations to cherish and enjoy.

The breathtaking vistas, lush forests, cascading waterfalls, and serene streams that greet you on your journey are not only beautiful but also fragile. As we explore and revel in the magnificence of these landscapes, it becomes our responsibility to act as custodians of nature, safeguarding its treasures for the long-term.

Preserving nature's treasures begins with respecting the delicate ecosystems that thrive in these environments. Staying on designated trails, leaving no trace of our presence, and avoiding disruptions to wildlife habitats are essential practices in maintaining the balance of these ecosystems.

Adopting sustainable practices during our hikes can significantly contribute to nature's preservation. By carrying reusable water bottles, disposing of waste responsibly, and minimizing our impact on the environment, we can help preserve the natural beauty of these landscapes for future generations.

Engaging in conservation efforts and supporting organizations dedicated to preserving natural habitats also plays a vital role. By donating to conservation initiatives and participating in restoration projects, we actively contribute to safeguarding the ecological health of the areas we explore.

Educating ourselves and others about the importance of preserving nature's treasures is a powerful way to inspire collective action. Sharing our experiences and raising awareness of the fragility of these environments encourages others to join in the effort to protect our planet's precious ecosystems.

Additionally, advocating for responsible environmental policies and supporting legislation that safeguards natural areas is crucial. By advocating for the protection of national parks, wildlife reserves, and natural heritage sites, we can ensure that these treasures remain intact for generations to come.

As we journey through the wonders of nature during our

"Scenic Hikes," let us be mindful of the impact we have on these landscapes. Embracing a mindset of preservation and sustainability allows us to savor nature's beauty while fulfilling our duty to safeguard its treasures.

By preserving nature's treasures today, we ensure that future generations can experience the same awe and wonder that we encounter during our explorations. Let us take up this responsibility with reverence and gratitude, cherishing the natural gifts that surround us and leaving a legacy of environmental stewardship for generations yet to come.

Community and Camaraderie

As you set forth on your "Scenic Hikes," you'll discover that these outdoor adventures provide not only an opportunity to connect with nature but also a chance to foster a sense of community and camaraderie among fellow hikers.

The trailhead becomes a meeting point where strangers with a shared love for nature come together, forming a diverse community of individuals seeking the same enriching experiences. Whether you're a seasoned hiker or a first timer, the trails welcome everyone with open arms, fostering a spirit of inclusivity and friendship.

As you traverse the paths, conversations flow effortlessly, and bonds are forged. Stories are exchanged, laughter echoes through the woods, and common experiences create a sense of unity among hikers from different walks of life.

During rest stops, you'll find hikers sharing snacks, offering trail tips, and providing encouragement to those embarking on challenging routes. The spirit of camaraderie flourishes as everyone becomes a part of a larger hiking family, bound by a shared passion for exploration.

Along the journey, trail companions become a source of motivation and support. The encouragement of fellow hikers can make even the steepest ascents feel conquerable, and the joy shared at reaching a scenic vista becomes even more rewarding in the company of newfound friends.

Beyond the immediate camaraderie on the trails, the hiking community extends to online forums, social media groups, and local clubs where hikers connect, share experiences, and plan future adventures together. These platforms provide a space to learn from each other, exchange valuable hiking insights, and inspire one another to explore new destinations.

The sense of community and camaraderie experienced during "Scenic Hikes" leaves an indelible mark, reminding us that the journey is not just about reaching a destination but also about connecting with the people we encounter along the way. The shared love for nature and the outdoors binds us together, transcending barriers and fostering a spirit of togetherness.

Whether hiking with friends, family, or kindred spirits you meet on the trail, the camaraderie experienced during these outdoor excursions enriches the journey and makes the memories all the more meaningful. So, as you lace up your hiking boots and set out on your adventures, embrace the opportunity to create lasting connections with fellow hikers, and relish in the sense of community that blooms amidst the beauty of nature.

Embracing the Journey

As you embark on your "Scenic Hikes," you'll quickly discover that the true essence of these adventures lies not just in reaching the destination but in fully embracing the journey itself.

Every step you take becomes an invitation to be present and attuned to the wonders around you. Each trail presents its own tapestry of sights, sounds, and sensations that beg to be savored. From the smallest wildflower to the grandest mountain peak, every aspect of nature's beauty calls for your attention and appreciation.

Embracing the journey means embracing the ebb and flow of the hike—the moments of uphill struggle and the smooth paths that lead you forward. It's about finding joy in the challenges and taking pride in the progress you make.

Pause to marvel at the intricate patterns of sunlight filtering through the forest canopy. Take a moment to listen to the symphony of bird calls that fill the air. Allow the gentle rustling of leaves to soothe your soul and the fragrance of the earth to awaken your senses.

Engage your curiosity and explore the hidden nooks and crannies along the trail. These unassuming places often reveal the most extraordinary surprises—a hidden waterfall, a serene pond, or a breathtaking view obscured by foliage.

Let go of time constraints and immerse yourself in the freedom of the natural world. Nature knows no schedules or deadlines, and in its embrace, you can release the burdens of daily life and reconnect with the simplicity of existence.

Throughout the journey, give yourself permission to be in awe of nature's majesty. Feel the humbling wonder as you stand beneath a towering waterfall or gaze out from a mountain summit. Allow yourself to feel a sense of oneness with the world around you.

Embracing the journey is about finding gratitude for every step you take and every experience you encounter. It's recognizing that each moment spent in nature is a gift—a chance to recharge, find peace, and be inspired.

As you trek through the breathtaking landscapes, take the time to be fully present, fully alive, and fully engaged in the adventure. For within the journey, you'll discover not only the beauty of nature but also the beauty within yourself—the strength, the resilience, and the wonder that make you a part of this grand tapestry of life.

So, let each footfall be a celebration of life, and each breath a testament to the vitality of existence. Embrace the journey in all its glory, and in doing so, you'll find that nature's embrace has the power to transform not only your hikes but also your heart and soul.

Hiking for All Levels

In the realm of "Scenic Hikes," there is a trail for every adventurer, regardless of their hiking experience or fitness level. This subsection celebrates the inclusivity of hiking, as it caters to both seasoned hikers seeking new challenges and beginners looking to embark on their first outdoor expedition.

For the avid hiker seeking adrenaline-pumping adventures, there are rugged trails that wind through challenging terrains, testing physical endurance and mental fortitude. These demanding paths lead to the most breathtaking vistas, rewarding hikers with awe-inspiring panoramas that make every effort worthwhile.

If you're new to hiking or prefer a more leisurely pace, fear not, for the trails of "Scenic Hikes" also welcome you with open arms. Gentle pathways weave through serene forests and alongside peaceful streams, allowing you to savor nature's beauty at a relaxed tempo.

The variety of trails ensures that everyone can find a hiking experience that suits their preferences and abilities. Moderate routes offer a balance between challenge and ease, providing a sense of accomplishment while allowing time to appreciate the scenery without feeling rushed.

Additionally, many trails are equipped with interpretive signs or guides that share fascinating insights into the natural history, flora, and fauna along the way. Such enriching experiences make hiking an educational journey, engaging both the mind and the body.

Moreover, some trails are accessible to individuals with mobility challenges, offering inclusive experiences that allow everyone to connect with nature's wonders. These paths may be paved or specially designed to accommodate wheelchairs and strollers, ensuring that nature's beauty is accessible to all.

Hiking for all levels fosters a sense of togetherness, as people of diverse backgrounds and abilities can share in the joy of exploring the great outdoors. Whether hiking alone, with friends, or in guided groups, the trails unite hikers with a common purpose—to immerse themselves in the splendor of nature.

So, whether you seek thrilling escapades, serene wanderings, or a bit of both, "Scenic Hikes" has a trail tailored for you. Embrace the opportunity to discover new facets of yourself and nature, as hiking for all levels creates an inclusive space where every hiker can find their place among the grand symphony of the great outdoors.

A Lifetime of Exploration

"Scenic Hikes" offers more than just a collection of trails; it presents an invitation to embark on a lifetime of exploration. Each hike becomes a chapter in a grand adventure, and the possibilities for discovery are endless.

As you venture through nature's wonders, you'll find that the desire to explore becomes insatiable. Each hike kindles a curiosity to seek out new trails, new landscapes, and new experiences. The allure of the unknown draws you forward, urging you to keep exploring and uncovering the hidden gems of the world.

Hiking becomes a lifelong journey, not bound by age or time. From the young-at-heart seniors to the youngest explorers, the trails cater to every stage of life. As the years pass, you'll come to realize that hiking isn't just an activity; it's a way of life—a path to keep learning, growing, and embracing the wonders of nature.

Through each season, the trails transform, revealing their unique beauty throughout the year. Spring carpets the forest floor with blossoms, summer paints the landscape in vibrant hues, autumn sets the trees ablaze with colors, and winter drapes everything in a pristine blanket of snow. A lifetime of exploration means experiencing nature's ever-changing tapestry in all its splendor.

Beyond the physical landscapes, hiking offers an exploration of the self. As you navigate the trails, you'll discover the strength of your body and mind. Each challenge you overcome becomes a testament to your resilience, and each breathtaking view becomes a reminder of the beauty that resides within you.

Hiking also fosters connections—with nature, with fellow adventurers, and with the world at large. Through shared experiences and encounters with diverse landscapes, you'll develop a deeper understanding of the interconnectedness of all life. The journey becomes a celebration of unity and a commitment to preserving the precious ecosystems that sustain us all.

With every hike, you leave a footprint—a mark of your presence on the trail and in the world. And just as nature leaves an impression on you, you, too, leave an imprint on the places you explore and the people you encounter.

A lifetime of exploration isn't confined to one region or one type of terrain. It spans continents, climates, and cultures. Whether you find yourself hiking along mountain ridges, traversing coastal paths, or meandering through meadows, each landscape offers its own wisdom and magic.

So, as you set out on your "Scenic Hikes," let each step be a celebration of a lifetime of exploration. Embrace the trails that unfold before you, and may each journey be a testament to the indomitable spirit of adventure that resides within us all. There is a world of wonders waiting to be discovered, and it begins with that first step into the heart of nature's embrace.

Conclusion

Scenic hikes are an ode to the beauty of the natural world and a celebration of our innate connection to the great outdoors. Through each step, we rediscover the wonder of existence and marvel at the intricate tapestry of life. So, put on your hiking boots, pack your sense of adventure, and allow "365 Fun Things to Do in Retirement" to be your guide to the most scenic trails and breathtaking landscapes. Embrace the joy of hiking, and with each step, let nature's symphony serenade your soul, igniting a profound appreciation for the beauty that surrounds us. The wonders of the world await your exploration – are you ready to embark on the scenic hikes of a lifetime?

CHAPTER 3: CREATIVE AND ARTISTIC PURSUITS

Painting and Drawing - Unlocking Your Artistic Side and Creating Unique Works of Art

Within the realm of "Scenic Hikes," lies a pathway to unlock your inner artist through the creative and meditative pursuit of painting and drawing. Embracing these artistic expressions allows you to capture the beauty of nature on canvas and paper, creating unique works of art that reflect your personal connection with the natural world.

As you hike through breathtaking landscapes, take the time to observe the play of light and shadow, the intricate details of flora, and the majesty of the vistas before you. Each step becomes an opportunity to absorb the nuances of the scenery, igniting a wellspring of inspiration for your artistic endeavors.

Painting and drawing provide a profound way to interpret nature's beauty through your unique perspective. With every brushstroke or pencil mark, you express your emotions, experiences, and perception of the world around you. The act of creating art becomes a form of meditation, allowing you to be fully present in the moment and immersed in the creative process.

You need not be a master artist to embark on this creative journey. Nature's canvas invites artists of all levels, from beginners to seasoned creators. Your art need not be a perfect representation; rather, it becomes a reflection of your individual connection with the landscapes that stir your soul.

Portable art supplies easily fit into a backpack, allowing you to set up your creative space amidst nature's grandeur. Under the open sky, let your imagination flow as you translate the beauty around you into strokes of color or lines on paper.

The creative process itself becomes a dialogue with nature. As you paint or sketch, you deepen your connection with the natural world, becoming attuned to the intricacies and subtleties of your surroundings. Through art, you cultivate a deeper appreciation for the wonders that surround you during your "Scenic Hikes."

Moreover, art serves as a timeless memento of your outdoor adventures. Each artwork becomes a keepsake, preserving the essence of the places you've explored and the memories you've forged. Whether you choose to frame your creations or compile them in a personal art journal, they become a cherished record of your journey through nature's gallery.

Painting and drawing on your "Scenic Hikes" go beyond mere

artistic expression; they become a celebration of your connection with the natural world. The canvas and paper become an extension of your heart, allowing you to share your love and reverence for nature through the medium of art.

So, as you embark on your creative and artistic pursuits during your hikes, remember that the process is as meaningful as the final creation. Embrace the joy of expressing yourself, capturing nature's beauty with each stroke, and allowing your artistic journey to deepen your connection with the landscapes that inspire you.

Writing and Storytelling - Sharing Personal Stories or Embarking on Imaginative Adventures with the Pen

Amidst the enchanting landscapes of "Scenic Hikes," a realm of storytelling and self-expression awaits, beckoning you to wield the power of the pen and unlock the wonders of writing. Whether you choose to share personal anecdotes or embark on imaginative adventures, writing becomes a cherished companion on your journey through nature's embrace.

As you traverse the trails, immerse yourself in the sensory experiences that nature offers. The rustling leaves, the whispering breeze, and the gentle babbling of streams become the backdrop for your creative exploration. Nature becomes the muse that fuels your words, igniting your creativity and inspiring stories waiting to be told.

For those who relish in recounting their personal experiences, writing becomes a way to capture the essence of each hike. You can journal your thoughts, emotions, and reflections, preserving the vivid memories of your outdoor escapades. In the pages of your journal, the details of each moment come alive, forming a narrative that intertwines with the landscapes you've encountered.

Moreover, writing offers a pathway to share the magic of nature with others. Through articles, blog posts, or social media, you can weave tales of the beauty and wonder found along your "Scenic Hikes," inviting readers to join you on your adventures from afar.

Alternatively, unleash your imagination and embark on literary quests through storytelling. Let the landscapes spark tales of mythical creatures roaming ancient forests or daring explorers on quests for hidden treasures. The canvas of nature becomes a boundless realm where your characters can roam, each trail offering a new chapter to their epic stories.

In the embrace of nature's beauty, writing becomes a meditative journey of self-discovery. Penning your thoughts allows you to delve deeper into your feelings and understand the profound impact nature has on your soul. Through writing, you can process your experiences, find clarity, and connect with the world more deeply.

Furthermore, the act of storytelling becomes a way to honor the landscapes that have inspired you. Your tales become a tribute to the majesty of mountains, the serenity of forests, and the tranquility of streams. With each word, you breathe life into the places you've explored, immortalizing them through the power of literature.

Writing and storytelling on your "Scenic Hikes" transcend the boundaries of time and space, carrying the essence of each journey into eternity. Through the written word, you become the author of your own adventures, crafting tales that intertwine with the wonders of nature. So, embrace the pen as your companion on the trails, and allow the art of writing to become an inseparable part of your journey through nature's timeless embrace.

Exploratory Photography - Capturing Special Moments and Enchanting Landscapes with the Camera

As you embark on your "Scenic Hikes," the art of exploratory photography presents itself as a delightful way to document your journey and immortalize the captivating moments and enchanting landscapes you encounter along the way.

With each step, you'll find yourself surrounded by breathtaking vistas, intricate details, and fleeting wonders. Exploratory

SERENA MITCHELL

photography becomes your lens to the world, allowing you to frame the beauty that unfolds before your eyes and seize the essence of each scene.

Through the lens of your camera, you become an artist, painting with light and shadow to create images that mirror the emotions and sensations awakened by nature. The play of sunlight on leaves, the dance of reflections in serene streams, and the interplay of colors in the sky become your palette, ready to be captured with every click.

Exploratory photography becomes an adventure of its own, as you seek out the perfect angles and compositions to encapsulate the magic of nature. The quest to find the ideal shot adds a new dimension to your hike, encouraging you to explore every nook and cranny for hidden gems and unique perspectives.

With your camera as your guide, you become an observer of the world around you, attuned to the tiniest details and the grandest vistas. Each photograph becomes a story, revealing the beauty and stories of the landscapes that grace your "Scenic Hikes."

Moreover, photography invites you to be fully present in the moment, to appreciate the fleeting nature of light, and to embrace the gift of the present. In the act of capturing a scene, you form a deep connection with the landscapes, acknowledging their ephemeral nature and the ever-changing canvas of nature's artistry.

The joy of exploratory photography lies not only in capturing the external beauty but also in reflecting the emotions and experiences you've encountered during your hike. Each photograph becomes a reflection of your personal journey, and the images you collect become cherished mementos that transport you back to the awe-inspiring moments of your outdoor adventures.

Exploratory photography transcends the limits of language, communicating the wonders of nature to others who might not have the opportunity to witness it firsthand. By sharing your photographs, you invite others to experience the beauty, tranquility, and grandeur of the landscapes you've explored.

As you journey through "Scenic Hikes," let your camera be an extension of your heart, capturing the essence of each step, each moment, and each breathtaking view. Embrace the magic of exploratory photography, for in each image lies a timeless testament to the wonders of the natural world and the adventure of your soul.

CHAPTER 4: FITNESS AND WELLNESS

Yoga and Meditation - Cultivating Mental Tranquility and Physical Well-being

In the realm of "Scenic Hikes," the path to inner peace and physical well-being is paved by the ancient practices of yoga and meditation. Amidst the natural splendor, yoga poses and meditation techniques become your allies in nurturing a harmonious connection between mind, body, and soul.

Yoga, a practice that unites movement and breath, becomes a moving meditation as you flow through asanas amidst the beauty of nature. Each pose becomes a graceful expression of strength and flexibility, and the rhythm of your breath weaves seamlessly with the gentle whispers of the wind.

The practice of yoga during your hikes allows you to stretch and strengthen your body while tuning into the present moment. With each inhale, you draw in the rejuvenating energy of the landscapes around you, and with each exhale, you release any tensions or worries that may have accompanied you on the journey.

As you move through the sequences, you'll find that the natural world becomes your sacred studio—a place of mindfulness where you can connect with the elements and the earth beneath your feet. With each pose, you ground yourself in the beauty of the surroundings, feeling a sense of oneness with nature.

Meditation, too, becomes a profound practice during your "Scenic Hikes." As you find a serene spot along the trail, you immerse yourself in meditation, silencing the chatter of the mind and embracing the stillness that nature offers. The rustling leaves and soft sounds of the wilderness become the backdrop for your inner journey.

Through meditation, you cultivate mental tranquility, finding refuge from the distractions of everyday life and finding solace in the present moment. The sights and sounds of nature become your anchors, grounding you in the here and now.

In the union of yoga and meditation, you discover a profound sense of wellness that permeates your being. The physical postures awaken vitality and energy, while meditation fosters clarity and peace of mind. Together, they become a harmonious duo, guiding you towards a state of holistic well-being.

Beyond the physical and mental benefits, the practice of yoga and meditation amidst nature serves as a reminder of the interconnectedness of all life. Your breath aligns with the rhythm of the earth, and your movements flow in harmony with the universe.

Incorporating yoga and meditation into your "Scenic Hikes" transforms your outdoor excursions into transformative journeys of self-discovery. As you cultivate mental tranquility and physical well-being, you deepen your connection with nature and nurture a profound appreciation for the sanctuary it offers to your mind, body, and soul.

Cycling Trips - Discovering New Routes and Enjoying Nature on Two Wheels

In the vast expanse of "Scenic Hikes," an exhilarating world of cycling trips unfolds, offering you the chance to explore nature's wonders on two wheels. As you pedal along winding trails and open roads, you'll discover a unique way to connect with the outdoors and experience the beauty of the landscapes in a thrilling and invigorating manner.

Cycling trips provide a fresh perspective on the natural world, allowing you to cover more ground and explore a greater range of terrain than on foot. The gentle breeze caresses your face as you ride, and the rhythmic motion of cycling becomes a liberating dance with nature.

As you venture along new routes, you'll uncover hidden gems and secret spots that are often missed by traditional hiking trails.

The thrill of discovery becomes a constant companion as each turn reveals new vistas, charming landscapes, and unexpected encounters with wildlife.

Cycling also offers a sense of freedom and fluidity, enabling you to embrace spontaneity and veer off the beaten path whenever a captivating sight captures your attention. With every twist and turn, you chart your own course, creating a journey that is uniquely yours.

Beyond the joy of exploration, cycling trips allow you to immerse yourself in the sights, sounds, and scents of nature. As you ride through lush forests, vibrant meadows, and tranquil waterways, you become a part of the natural symphony, harmonizing with the rhythms of the environment.

The physical benefits of cycling are abundant, as the activity strengthens your cardiovascular system, tones muscles, and enhances overall fitness. Yet, the rewards extend far beyond the physical. Cycling in nature nourishes your spirit and invigorates your mind, leaving you with a profound sense of well-being and contentment.

Whether you embark on leisurely rides, adrenaline-pumping mountain biking, or serene road cycling, each cycling trip becomes an opportunity to reconnect with the world around you. As the wheels turn, your senses come alive, and the beauty of nature becomes an ever-changing tapestry that surrounds you.

During your "Scenic Hikes," let cycling become a cherished addition to your repertoire of outdoor adventures. Embrace the freedom of the open road, the thrill of discovery, and the exhilaration of being in sync with the pulse of nature on two wheels. Cycling trips become a celebration of movement and connection—a delightful way to savor the beauty of the landscapes and revel in the sheer joy of experiencing nature's embrace.

Water Activities - Swimming, Rowing, and Kayaking to Stay Fit and Have Fun

In the realm of "Scenic Hikes," the wonders of water beckon with an array of invigorating activities that keep you fit and introduce you to a world of aquatic adventure. Embrace the refreshing embrace of the waters as you engage in swimming, rowing, and kayaking, unlocking the joy of staying active while immersed in the beauty of nature's aquatic treasures.

Swimming becomes a delightful way to merge with nature's watery realms. Whether in serene lakes, tranquil ponds, or crystal-clear rivers, the waters invite you to dive in and experience a sense of weightlessness. As you glide through the water, you'll feel a liberating sense of freedom, and the rhythmic strokes become a meditative dance with the currents.

Rowing presents a delightful activity that combines physical exertion with the gentle serenity of nature. Setting sail on calm waters, you become the captain of your journey, guiding the boat through peaceful lakes or meandering rivers. With each oar stroke, you forge a connection with the water, propelling yourself forward amidst the tranquility of the surroundings.

Kayaking offers a thrilling escapade that enables you to explore hidden coves, navigate through winding waterways, and encounter the untouched beauty of nature. Paddling your kayak, you become an intrepid explorer, gliding through picturesque landscapes and discovering the rich diversity of aquatic ecosystems.

Beyond the joy of recreation, water activities bestow numerous health benefits. Swimming, rowing, and kayaking are excellent full-body workouts that engage various muscle groups, strengthen the cardiovascular system, and promote overall fitness. The low-impact nature of these activities makes them accessible to individuals of all ages and fitness levels, fostering a sense of well-being and vitality.

As you immerse yourself in water activities during your "Scenic Hikes," you'll find that the aquatic realm becomes a source of rejuvenation for the body, mind, and soul. The gentle ripples of water serve as a soothing soundtrack, and the shimmering reflections of sunlight on the surface evoke a sense of tranquility.

Moreover, water activities allow you to witness nature from a unique perspective. From the vantage point of the water, you'll encounter wildlife, aquatic plants, and captivating landscapes that are often hidden from view. These close encounters with nature's aquatic wonders deepen your connection with the natural world.

Embrace the allure of water activities during your outdoor adventures, and let the waters become a portal to both fitness and fun. As you swim, row, or kayak through the scenic waters, revel in the enchantment of being part of nature's aquatic symphony. The joyful splashes, the gentle currents, and the breathtaking vistas become the backdrop for memorable moments that will stay with you long after you've left the water's embrace.

CHAPTER 5: TRAVEL AND

GLOBAL ADVENTURES

Slow Travel: Exploring New Destinations with a Sense of Curiosity and Calmness

In a fast-paced world, where time seems to slip through our fingers, slow travel offers a refreshing and enriching alternative for retirees seeking to immerse themselves in the beauty of new destinations. Unlike the hurried itineraries of traditional tourism, slow travel invites explorers to savor each moment, connect with local cultures, and forge meaningful experiences. In this subsection, we delve into the art of slow travel and how it can transform your retirement adventures.

Embracing a Mindful Journey: Slow travel is not just about the destination; it's about embracing the journey itself. When you embark on a slow travel experience, you allow yourself to be fully present in each moment, savoring the little details that might otherwise go unnoticed. From the taste of local delicacies to the laughter shared with newfound friends, mindful travel provides a profound sense of gratification and fulfillment.

Discovering Off-the-Beaten-Path Gems: One of the joys of slow travel is the opportunity to wander off the beaten path and discover hidden gems that escape the average tourist's eye. Whether it's a secluded village nestled in a picturesque valley, or an ancient temple tucked away in the heart of a bustling city, these unexplored wonders can leave a lasting imprint on your soul.

Immerse Yourself in local Cultures: Rather than observing from a distance, slow travel encourages you to actively engage with the local culture. Interact with friendly locals, participate in traditional festivities, and learn about the customs that define a community's identity. Through these authentic experiences, you gain a deeper appreciation for the world's diversity and the richness of human connections.

Relish in the Joy of Slowing Down: In a world that rushes from one place to another, slow travel teaches us the art of slowing down. It's an opportunity to break free from the constraints of schedules and deadlines, giving yourself permission to take detours, linger in charming cafes, and relish in moments of tranquility. By embracing a more leisurely pace, you'll find that time expands, and each experience becomes more meaningful.

Mindful Packing and Sustainable Choices: Slow travel also aligns with a mindset of sustainable and mindful living. Pack light and consciously choose eco-friendly accommodation and transportation options. Reduce your environmental footprint while supporting businesses that prioritize responsible practices. By being mindful of our impact as travelers, we contribute to the preservation of natural wonders and cultural heritage for future generations.

Creating Lasting Memories: When you embrace slow travel, you're not collecting passport stamps; you're creating cherished memories that will stay with you forever. These are the kind of memories that you'll share with loved ones around the dinner table or in a cozy gathering, reminiscing about the extraordinary experiences that enriched your retirement journey.

Slow travel is an invitation to step off the conveyor belt of mass tourism and approach your travels with a fresh perspective. With curiosity as your compass and calmness as your companion, you'll find that the essence of each destination reveals itself in ways you never imagined. So, open your heart to the beauty of slow travel, and let the world unveil its wonders at your own pace.

Road trips: experiencing the allure of adventures on the open road and visiting unique places

Few experiences embody the spirit of freedom and adventure like a road trip. The open road beckons, promising a thrilling journey of exploration and the chance to uncover hidden treasures along the way. In this subsection, we dive into the art of road trips, offering insights into planning unforgettable adventures and discovering the magic of unique places.

Embrace the Journey, not just the Destination! Road trips are as much about the journey as they are about the destination. Embrace the spontaneity of the open road and be open to unexpected detours that lead to surprising discoveries. While having a rough itinerary is helpful, leave room for serendipity and allow yourself to follow your instincts and curiosity.

Choose Your Ideal Route: The beauty of a road trip lies in the freedom to choose your route. Opt for scenic byways, wind through majestic mountain passes, or cruise along coastal roads with breathtaking ocean views. Tailor your route to your preferences, whether it's exploring national parks, historic landmarks, charming small towns, or vibrant cities.

Pack Essentials for Comfort and Safety: As you embark on your road trip, make sure to pack essentials for comfort and safety. Comfortable clothing, snacks, water, and a first aid kit are essential companions. Don't forget to carry a roadmap or a GPS device to ensure you stay on track and avoid getting lost.

Immersive Pit Stops: The charm of road trips lies in the delightful pit stops you encounter along the way. These can be quirky roadside attractions, family-owned diners serving up local delicacies, or awe-inspiring natural wonders. Embrace the joy of exploring these offbeat spots, as they often become some of the most cherished memories of your journey.

Embrace Camping Adventures: For an authentic road trip experience, consider camping at scenic locations along your route. Sleeping under the stars and waking up to the sounds of nature heightens your connection with the landscapes you traverse. Whether it's in a national park or a remote wilderness area, camping adds a touch of adventure and nostalgia to your journey.

Capture Moments and Create Memories: A road trip is a visual feast of landscapes, landmarks, and unforgettable moments. Take the time to capture these memories through photographs and videos, documenting the highlights of your adventure. These mementos will become treasured souvenirs, allowing you to relive the magic of your road trip long after it's over.

Embrace Flexibility and Patience: While road trips offer incredible freedom, they also require flexibility and patience. Weather conditions, unexpected road closures, or other unforeseen events may necessitate changes to your plans. Embrace these moments as part of the adventure and view them as opportunities for new experiences.

Share the Road with Companions: A road trip becomes even more memorable when shared with friends, family, or like-minded companions. Consider embarking on this journey together, sharing laughter, stories, and the joy of exploration. The bonds forged during a road trip often last a lifetime.

Road trips are more than just a mode of transportation; they are journeys of self-discovery and wonder. Each mile brings the thrill of anticipation and the promise of new experiences. So, gather your spirit of adventure, hit the open road, and let the allure of road trips lead you to the magic of unique places waiting to be explored.

Travel Volunteering: Giving Meaning to Retirement by Helping Communities Worldwide

Retirement marks a chapter in life where the pursuit of personal fulfillment takes center stage. One immensely rewarding way to add purpose and meaning to your golden years is through travel volunteering. In this subsection, we explore the transformative power of travel volunteering, where retirees can use their time, skills, and compassion to make a positive impact on communities around the world.

The Joy of Giving Back: Travel volunteering offers a unique opportunity to give back to society and make a real difference in the lives of others. By dedicating your time and expertise, you can contribute to projects that support education, healthcare, environmental conservation, community development, and more. The fulfillment derived from helping others is immeasurable and can foster a profound sense of purpose in your retirement journey.

Choosing the Right Volunteering Project: When considering travel volunteering opportunities, carefully choose a project that aligns with your interests and skills. Whether teaching English to local children, participating in wildlife conservation efforts, or assisting in sustainable farming practices, finding a project that resonates with you ensures a meaningful and rewarding experience.

Engaging Cultural Exchange: Travel volunteering is not just about offering assistance; it's also about engaging in cross-cultural exchange. Embrace the chance to immerse yourself in the customs, traditions, and daily life of the communities you serve. In return, you'll gain a deeper understanding of global perspectives and cultivate empathy and respect for diverse cultures.

Sustainable and Responsible Volunteering: Prioritize sustainable and responsible volunteering practices to ensure your efforts have a positive and lasting impact. Collaborate with reputable organizations that prioritize community-driven projects and follow ethical guidelines. Sustainability involves empowering locals with the skills and resources needed to maintain and expand the initiatives you support.

Gaining New Perspectives and Lifelong Memories: Travel volunteering introduces you to unique and enriching experiences that leave lasting impressions. You'll forge meaningful connections with fellow volunteers, locals, and the people you help, creating cherished memories that will stay with you forever. These memories become part of your life story, enriching the tapestry of your retirement years.

Personal Growth and Lifelong Learning

Beyond the impact on the communities you serve, travel volunteering also fosters personal growth and lifelong learning. It challenges you to adapt to new environments, work collaboratively with diverse teams, and tackle unexpected situations. The skills and insights gained during your volunteering journey can have a positive ripple effect in all aspects of your life.

Making Retirement Travel Meaningful: Incorporating travel volunteering into your retirement adventures allows you to experience the world in a deeper and more meaningful way. Rather than merely sightseeing, you'll engage with locals and make a lasting impact, leaving behind a legacy of compassion and support.

Connecting with Like-Minded Souls: Travel volunteering attracts like-minded individuals from around the globe who share a passion for making a difference. The friendships formed with fellow volunteers can be profound, creating a network of people who share a common purpose and vision for a better world.

Incorporating travel volunteering into your retirement journey is an invitation to channel your time and energy toward making the world a better place. By helping communities and fostering cross-cultural understanding, you'll find that your retirement gains new significance and becomes a time of purpose, connection, and global impact.

CHAPTER 6: COOKING AND GASTRONOMY

Cooking Classes - Experimenting with New Recipes and Improving Culinary Skills

Food has the remarkable ability to bring people together and create unforgettable experiences. In this chapter, we delve into the delightful world of cooking and gastronomy, focusing on the joy of attending cooking classes during retirement. These classes provide an excellent opportunity to explore new recipes, enhance culinary skills, and savor the pleasure of creating delectable dishes.

The Pleasures of Culinary Education: Retirement opens up a world of possibilities, and for those with a passion for food, cooking classes offer a chance to embark on an exciting culinary journey. Whether you're a seasoned home cook or a complete novice in the kitchen, these classes cater to all skill levels and provide a supportive and engaging environment to learn and grow.

Finding the Perfect Class: Cooking classes come in various formats, from one-day workshops to comprehensive multi-week courses.

Start by researching local culinary schools, community centers, or cooking academies that offer classes tailored to your interests. Some schools specialize in specific cuisines, such as Italian, French, or Asian, while others focus on techniques like baking, grilling, or pastry making. Choose a class that aligns with your preferences and culinary goals.

Embrace New Cuisines: One of the most exciting aspects of cooking classes is the opportunity to explore and master new cuisines from around the world. Step out of your comfort zone and immerse yourself in the flavors of different cultures. Whether it's learning to make traditional sushi, crafting the perfect Spanish paella, or experimenting with the spices of Indian cuisine, each class will broaden your culinary horizons.

Hands-On Learning: Cooking is an art best learned through practice, and cooking classes prioritize hands-on experience. As you work side by side with professional chefs or experienced instructors, you'll gain valuable insights, tips, and techniques that will elevate your cooking abilities. From knife skills to precise seasoning, the guidance of a knowledgeable mentor will boost your confidence in the kitchen.

Teamwork and Socializing: Cooking classes provide a fantastic opportunity to socialize and make new friends with similar interests. You'll likely collaborate with other participants during group activities, fostering a sense of camaraderie and shared passion for food. Bonding over the preparation and enjoyment of a delicious meal creates lasting memories and meaningful connections.

Bringing the Experience Home: As you experiment with new recipes and techniques, remember that the knowledge gained in cooking classes is meant to be shared. Invite friends and family over for a special dinner where you can showcase your newfound culinary expertise. Cooking becomes even more rewarding when you can bring joy to others through your delicious creations.

Conclusion

Cooking classes offer an enriching and fulfilling experience during retirement, allowing you to nurture your love for food while enhancing your culinary skills. The journey of exploring new recipes, learning from experienced chefs, and savoring the results of your efforts is a truly satisfying adventure. Embrace the art of cooking, and let it become a delightful part of your retirement lifestyle, bringing joy and togetherness to every meal you prepare. So put on your apron, pick up your utensils, and get ready to create culinary masterpieces that will leave a lasting impression on your taste buds and your heart. Buon appetito!

Food and Wine Tours - Discovering Regional Flavors and Traditions through Tastings and Culinary Experiences

For the epicurean retirees and wine enthusiasts, few experiences rival the joy of embarking on food and wine tours during retirement. These tours provide a unique opportunity to explore the culinary delights of different regions, savor authentic dishes, and indulge in the world of exquisite wines. In this subsection, we delve into the pleasures of food and wine tours and how they can add a delectable touch to your retirement adventures.

Immerse Yourself in Culinary Heritage: Food and wine tours are a gateway to the heart and soul of a region's culinary heritage. Whether you're touring the vineyards of Tuscany, the vine-laden valleys of Napa, or the picturesque wineries of Bordeaux, each destination offers a captivating glimpse into its local flavors and traditions. From artisanal cheeses and charcuterie to farm-fresh produce and tantalizing pastries, every bite tells a story deeply rooted in the region's history and culture.

Guided Tastings and Culinary Experiences: One of the highlights of food and wine tours is the chance to participate in guided tastings and culinary experiences. Accompanied by knowledgeable sommeliers and food experts, you'll learn the art of wine tasting, appreciating the subtle nuances of different vintages, and pairing them harmoniously with delectable dishes. The experience is not just about the flavors but also about understanding the craftsmanship and dedication that go into creating these culinary masterpieces.

Discover Hidden Gems: Food and wine tours often take you

off the beaten path, leading you to hidden culinary gems that might otherwise remain undiscovered. These hidden gems could be family-run trattorias, charming bistros, or small boutique wineries that offer unparalleled authenticity and charm. Exploring these lesser-known establishments brings a sense of adventure and an element of surprise to your gastronomic journey.

Connect with Local Artisans: In addition to tasting exquisite food and wine, food and wine tours offer the chance to meet the passionate artisans behind these creations. Engaging with local winemakers, chefs, and producers allows you to gain insights into their time-honored techniques and their dedication to preserving culinary traditions. These encounters add a personal touch to your experiences and create lasting memories.

Culinary Workshops and Cooking Demos: Some food and wine tours go beyond tastings and incorporate culinary workshops and cooking demonstrations. Participating in hands-on cooking classes led by skilled chefs allows you to learn how to recreate regional dishes back home. These newfound culinary skills can become treasured souvenirs that you can share with loved ones and enjoy long after the tour has ended.

Conclusion

Food and wine tours offer an unforgettable culinary expedition during retirement, inviting you to explore regional flavors, traditions, and the art of winemaking. With each tasting and culinary experience, you'll discover the rich tapestry of a region's culinary heritage, expanding your appreciation for the diversity and creativity of the culinary world. These tours are an indulgent way to celebrate life's pleasures and create cherished memories that will leave a lingering taste of joy and satisfaction. So, raise your glass and savor the culinary wonders that await you on your food and wine tour, celebrating the delightful fusion of food, wine, and culture. Salute!

Gardening an Edible Garden - Cultivating Fresh Fruits and Vegetables for a Healthy and Sustainable Diet

For retirees with a passion for nature and a desire to lead a healthy lifestyle, gardening an edible garden offers a fulfilling and rewarding experience. This subsection delves into the joys of growing your own fruits and vegetables, embracing sustainable practices, and enjoying the delectable rewards of your labor while fostering a deeper connection with nature.

The Pleasures of Edible Gardening: An edible garden is a source of endless delight, providing a sense of accomplishment as you nurture and witness the growth of your plants from seeds to harvest. There's a unique satisfaction in knowing that the fresh produce you enjoy on your plate comes directly from your own backyard. Engaging in gardening activities offers therapeutic benefits, such as reducing stress, improving mood, and fostering a sense of purpose during retirement.

Choosing the Right Location: Selecting the ideal location for your edible garden is crucial for its success. Look for a spot in your yard that receives ample sunlight throughout the day and has good drainage. If space is limited, consider vertical gardening or utilizing containers to grow your favorite fruits and vegetables. This allows you to maximize the available area and create a lush and productive garden even in small spaces.

Cultivating a Diverse Range of Produce: One of the exciting aspects of edible gardening is the opportunity to cultivate a diverse range of fruits and vegetables. Tailor your garden to include your favorite seasonal produce, as well as experimenting with unique and heirloom varieties. Whether it's juicy tomatoes, crisp lettuce, vibrant bell peppers, or luscious strawberries, each harvest promises a bounty of fresh flavors.

Embracing Sustainable Practices: Edible gardening aligns with sustainability principles, allowing you to reduce your carbon footprint and contribute to a healthier environment. Implementing eco-friendly practices, such as composting kitchen scraps for nutrient-rich soil, using natural pest control methods, and collecting rainwater for irrigation, helps create a garden that thrives harmoniously with nature.

Nurturing a Connection with Nature: Gardening offers a unique opportunity to connect with nature on a deeper level. As you tend to your plants, you'll become attuned to the changing seasons and the intricacies of the natural world. Observing pollinators buzzing around your flowers and seeing the cycle of life in your garden fosters a profound appreciation for the beauty and interconnectedness of all living things.

Sharing the Harvest: An abundant edible garden often yields more produce than you can consume alone. Embrace the joy of sharing your harvest with friends, family, and neighbors, spreading the benefits of your gardening endeavors beyond your own table. Consider participating in local farmers' markets or food donation programs, contributing to your community's well-being and food security.

Conclusion

Gardening an edible garden is a deeply enriching and sustainable endeavor during retirement, allowing you to cultivate fresh, nutritious produce while fostering a stronger connection with the natural world. Through this rewarding practice, you'll not only enjoy the physical benefits of a healthy diet but also experience the mental and emotional rewards of nurturing and witnessing the growth of your garden. As you embrace the cycles of nature and savor the delicious fruits of your labor, you'll find that gardening an edible garden is a nourishing and life-enriching journey that

SERENA MITCHELL

can be cherished for years to come. Happy gardening!

CHAPTER 7: DIY PROJECTS AND CRAFTS

DIY Crafts - Creating Handmade Items to Decorate the Home or Gift to Loved Ones

In the fast-paced digital age, there's something uniquely satisfying about engaging in do-it-yourself (DIY) crafts and creating handmade items. For retirees with a penchant for creativity and a desire to add a personal touch to their living spaces or gifts for loved ones, this subsection explores the joys of DIY crafts. Whether you're a seasoned crafter or a beginner looking to explore your artistic side, DIY crafts offer a fulfilling and meaningful way to express yourself and craft cherished keepsakes.

Embracing the Joy of Crafting: DIY crafts are more than just a creative outlet; they offer a meditative and fulfilling experience. Engaging in hands-on crafting activities provides a sense of accomplishment as you transform raw materials into beautiful and functional pieces. The process of crafting itself becomes a therapeutic journey that allows you to unwind and escape the hustle and bustle of everyday life.

Creating Personalized Home Décor: One of the delights of DIY crafts is the ability to personalize your home decor. From handmade wall art and decorative pillows to intricately designed picture frames and unique centerpieces, each crafted piece infuses your living space with warmth and character. DIY home decor reflects your individual style and tells a story that is uniquely yours.

Handmade Gifts from the Heart: DIY crafts offer the perfect opportunity to create thoughtful and heartfelt gifts for your loved ones. Handmade presents convey the effort and love put into crafting each item, making them cherished keepsakes for the recipients. Whether it's a hand-knitted scarf, a custom-made photo album, or a hand-painted mug, these gifts become precious reminders of the special bond shared with family and friends.

Exploring Various Crafting Techniques: DIY crafts encompass a wide array of crafting techniques that cater to various interests and skill levels. From knitting and crochet to woodworking, sewing, and paper crafting, there's a craft suited for every retiree's passion and expertise. The abundance of crafting tutorials and resources available online and in local crafting communities makes it easy to learn new techniques and expand your creative repertoire.

Sustainable and Eco-Friendly Crafting: Embracing DIY crafts can also align with sustainability principles, as you have control over the materials used in your projects. Consider repurposing old or discarded items into new creations, reducing waste and contributing to an eco-friendlier lifestyle. Crafting with natural, biodegradable, or recycled materials adds an extra layer of satisfaction to your DIY endeavors.

Crafting as a Social Activity: Crafting need not be a solitary pursuit; it can also be a wonderful social activity. Join local crafting groups or invite friends over for crafting sessions to share ideas, inspiration, and camaraderie. Crafting together fosters a sense of community and provides opportunities for learning from others' experiences and skills.

Conclusion

DIY crafts offer a fulfilling and expressive outlet for retirees to unleash their creativity and craft unique and meaningful items for their homes and loved ones. Engaging in hands-on crafting activities allows you to infuse your living spaces with personal touches and create heartfelt gifts that will be treasured for years to come. As you explore various crafting techniques and immerse yourself in the joy of making, you'll discover that DIY crafts are not just about creating tangible items but also about nurturing your soul and embracing the beauty of handmade artistry. So, gather your crafting supplies, let your imagination soar, and embark on a creative journey that will add beauty, love, and warmth to your life during retirement. Happy crafting!

Woodworking - Learning Woodworking Skills and Crafting Unique and Functional Objects

Woodworking is an age-old craft that offers retirees a wonderful opportunity to engage in a hands-on and rewarding hobby. Whether you're an experienced woodworker or a beginner looking to learn new skills, this subsection explores the joys of woodworking and the satisfaction of crafting unique and functional objects from this versatile and beautiful material.

The Artistry of Woodworking: Woodworking is a true art form, allowing retirees to transform raw pieces of wood into beautifully crafted objects. From intricately carved designs to smoothly polished surfaces, each woodworking project showcases the skill and creativity of the craftsman. Engaging in woodworking not only yields functional pieces but also creates lasting works of art to be admired and appreciated.

Exploring Various Woodworking Techniques: Woodworking offers a wide array of techniques, catering to different interests and skill levels. Beginners can start with simple projects like building basic shelves or picture frames, while seasoned woodworkers can take on more complex endeavors, such as crafting furniture, cabinets, or even sculptures. Learning and mastering these techniques allows retirees to continually challenge themselves and take their craftsmanship to new heights.

Crafting Unique and Customized Items: One of the delights of woodworking is the ability to create customized and one-of-a-kind pieces. Whether it's a handcrafted wooden jewelry box, a personalized cutting board, or a bespoke rocking chair, each item reflects the maker's unique style and preferences. Woodworking empowers retirees to craft objects that perfectly fit their needs and showcase their creativity.

A Sustainable and Eco-Friendly Hobby: Woodworking can be a sustainable and eco-friendly hobby, especially when using reclaimed or responsibly sourced wood. Upcycling old furniture or salvaging wood from discarded items reduces waste and contributes to a more environmentally conscious lifestyle. By giving new life to wood that might otherwise be discarded, woodworkers participate in a meaningful form of recycling and conservation.

Engaging the Mind and Body: Engaging in woodworking exercises both the mind and body, offering a holistic and satisfying experience. The process of planning and designing a project hones problem-solving skills, while the physical act of sawing, carving, and sanding provides an excellent form of exercise. Woodworking can be meditative and therapeutic, helping retirees maintain mental acuity and overall well-being.

Joining Woodworking Communities: Woodworking is a hobby that fosters a strong sense of community. Joining local woodworking clubs or online forums allows retirees to connect with fellow enthusiasts, share tips, and exchange ideas. The support and camaraderie of the woodworking community add to the enjoyment of the craft and provide opportunities for lifelong learning and inspiration.

Conclusion

Woodworking is a fulfilling and creative hobby that allows retirees to master woodworking skills and craft unique and functional objects. Whether creating simple home decor pieces or intricate furniture, each woodworking project is a testament to the artisan's craftsmanship and creativity. Engaging in this age-old craft provides a meditative and rewarding experience, where retirees can immerse themselves in the art of transforming wood into timeless and cherished objects. As you explore various woodworking techniques and create with your own hands, you'll discover the joy of bringing beautiful and functional creations to life. So, pick up your tools, embrace the artistry of woodworking, and embark on a journey of creativity and self-expression that will leave a lasting legacy for generations to come. Happy woodworking!

Recycled Crafts - Transforming Salvage Materials into Eco-Friendly Art Pieces

Recycled crafts offer retirees a unique and eco-conscious way to unleash their creativity while making a positive impact on the environment. This subsection explores the joys of transforming salvage materials into beautiful and eco-friendly art pieces. From upcycling discarded items to repurposing old materials, recycled crafts not only showcase ingenuity but also contribute to a sustainable and greener lifestyle.

The Beauty of Repurposing: Recycled crafts celebrate the beauty of repurposing materials that might otherwise end up in landfills. Retirees can breathe new life into old and forgotten items, giving them a fresh purpose and identity. Whether it's using old jars to create charming candle holders or turning scrap wood into decorative wall art, each recycled craft project highlights the artistry of transformation.

Exploring Salvage Materials: The possibilities for recycled crafts are virtually limitless, as salvage materials can include a wide range of items like glass bottles, tin cans, cardboard, fabrics, and more. Retirees can let their imaginations run wild, experimenting with various materials and exploring innovative ways to incorporate them into their artistic creations.

Fostering Eco-Friendly Practices: Engaging in recycled crafts aligns with eco-friendly principles, as it reduces waste and minimizes the consumption of new resources. By utilizing salvage materials, retirees actively participate in the sustainable movement, contributing to a healthier and cleaner environment. Recycling materials for creative purposes also sets an example for others to follow, inspiring more people to embrace environmentally responsible practices.

Unique and Artistic Expressions: Recycled crafts offer retirees the opportunity to showcase their unique artistic expressions. Each piece crafted from salvage materials becomes a distinct and one-of-a-kind creation. From colorful mosaic art made from broken tiles to whimsical sculptures assembled from scrap metal, recycled crafts embody the individuality of the artist and the beauty of imperfection.

A Source of Inspiration: Recycled crafts encourage resourcefulness and inspire creative problem-solving. As retirees brainstorm ideas for their projects, they develop a keen eye for spotting potential in discarded items and finding innovative ways to incorporate them into their artwork. This resourcefulness carries over into other aspects of life, fostering a mindset of sustainability and ingenuity.

Connecting with the Green Community: Recycled crafts often intersect with a passionate and like-minded community that values sustainability and creativity. Retirees can join local crafting groups or online platforms that focus on eco-friendly art and upcycling. Engaging with fellow green enthusiasts not only provides inspiration but also opens doors to new friendships and opportunities for collaborative projects.

Conclusion

Recycled crafts offer retirees a chance to channel their artistic flair while making a positive impact on the environment. Transforming salvage materials into eco-friendly art pieces showcases the ingenuity and resourcefulness of the artist and contributes to a more sustainable way of living. Engaging in recycled crafts is not just about creating art; it's a meaningful way to express care for the planet and inspire others to embrace a greener lifestyle. So gather your salvaged materials, let your creativity flow, and embark on a journey of turning discarded items into beautiful and environmentally conscious art pieces. Happy crafting!

CHAPTER 8: CULTURAL EXPERIENCES

Theater and Performances - Enjoying Plays, Concerts, and Artistic Performances

Immersing oneself in the world of theater and live performances is a vibrant and enriching way for retirees to embrace cultural experiences. In this subsection, we explore the joy of attending plays, concerts, and various artistic performances. Whether relishing classic theater productions, savoring the sounds of live music, or witnessing captivating dance performances, cultural experiences offer retirees the chance to be captivated by the arts and celebrate the beauty of human expression.

The Magic of Live Theater: Live theater has a captivating allure that transports audiences into captivating narratives and mesmerizing performances. Whether it's witnessing a classic Shakespearean play, a modern drama, or a delightful musical, the intimacy and immediacy of live theater create a unique and immersive experience. The raw emotions and energy of the actors bring stories to life, leaving a lasting impact on those who partake in these performances.

Savoring the Sounds of Live Music: Attending live concerts is a treat for the senses, as retirees immerse themselves in the magic of music. From symphony orchestras playing classical masterpieces to contemporary bands performing modern hits, live music performances offer a wide range of genres to suit diverse musical tastes. The shared experience of being surrounded by fellow music enthusiasts enhances the joy of the performance.

The Artistry of Artistic Performances: Artistic performances encompass a plethora of creative expressions, such as dance recitals, opera, ballet, circus acts, and more. Witnessing the mastery of talented performers gracefully moving across the stage or executing daring acrobatics is a testament to the beauty and skill of human artistry. Artistic performances celebrate the diversity and ingenuity of the performing arts, leaving spectators in awe of the spectacle before them.

Supporting Local Talent and Culture: Cultural experiences provide the opportunity to support local talent and cultural institutions within the community. By attending local theater productions, concerts, and performances, retirees actively contribute to the thriving arts scene in their area. This support nurtures creativity and fosters an appreciation for the cultural heritage of the region.

Lifelong Learning and Enrichment: Cultural experiences serve as a form of lifelong learning and enrichment. They offer retirees the chance to broaden their horizons, gain insights into different cultures and historical periods, and develop a deeper appreciation for the arts. Attending workshops, lectures, and post-performance discussions enhances the experience, providing additional context and understanding of the artistic works.

Social Engagement and Connection: Participating in cultural experiences is a wonderful way to engage socially with like-minded individuals who share a passion for the arts. Attending performances with friends or joining cultural clubs and organizations fosters connections and friendships centered around shared interests. The collective experience of savoring cultural delights strengthens bonds and enriches social life during retirement.

Conclusion

Cultural experiences, such as theater performances, concerts, and artistic displays, open a world of inspiration and wonder for retirees. By immersing themselves in live performances and celebrating the beauty of human expression, retirees can enrich their lives with art, music, and the magic of storytelling. Engaging in cultural experiences offers a dynamic and invigorating way to celebrate the arts, support local talent, and foster a deep appreciation for the diversity of human creativity. So, step into the world of cultural enchantment, embrace the performing arts, and let the power of artistic expression uplift your spirit and bring joy to your retirement journey.

Book Clubs and Reading Groups - Engaging with Other Book Enthusiasts to Discuss and Share Ideas

For retirees who have a passion for literature and a desire to explore the world of books, joining a book club or reading group offers a delightful and intellectually stimulating experience. This subsection delves into the joys of book clubs and reading groups, where retirees can connect with fellow book enthusiasts, engage in lively discussions, and share their love for literature.

The Pleasure of Shared Reading: Book clubs and reading groups provide the pleasure of shared reading experiences. Participants collectively select a book to read, allowing everyone to delve into the same literary world and embark on literary journeys together. The shared reading experience creates a sense of camaraderie and fosters a deeper appreciation for the chosen books.

Diverse Reading Selections: One of the delights of book clubs and reading groups is the diversity of reading selections. Members often take turns suggesting books, leading to a varied and eclectic mix of genres and authors. Exploring a wide range of literature exposes retirees to new perspectives, genres, and writing styles, expanding their literary horizons.

Engaging Discussions and Exchange of Ideas: Book club meetings are opportunities for retirees to engage in thought-provoking discussions about the books they've read. Sharing insights, interpretations, and emotional responses to the stories enriches the reading experience and allows members to gain deeper understandings of the books. These discussions often lead to new perspectives and interpretations that may not have occurred to individual readers.

Building Lifelong Friendships: Participating in book clubs and reading groups nurtures connections and fosters new friendships. Common interests in literature provide a strong foundation for meaningful conversations and shared experiences. The shared passion for books creates a supportive and welcoming environment where retirees can develop lasting friendships with like-minded individuals.

Stimulating the Mind: Engaging in regular book discussions stimulates the mind and keeps cognitive abilities sharp during retirement. Analyzing characters, plotlines, and themes exercises critical thinking skills, while articulating thoughts during discussions hones communication and public speaking abilities. These intellectual exercises contribute to mental acuity and mental well-being.

Flexibility and Adaptability: Book clubs and reading groups offer flexibility, allowing retirees to choose the level of commitment that suits their preferences. Some groups may meet monthly, while others meet more or less frequently. Virtual book clubs also offer the opportunity to connect with book enthusiasts worldwide, transcending geographical boundaries and fostering a global community of readers.

Conclusion

Book clubs and reading groups provide retirees with an exciting and engaging way to explore literature, connect with fellow book lovers, and stimulate intellectual discussions. The shared reading experiences, diverse selections, and lively conversations create an enriching and enjoyable literary journey. Engaging in book club discussions allows retirees to delve deeper into the worlds of books, gaining fresh perspectives and forging new friendships along the way. So, pick up your favorite book, join a book club, and let the magic of shared reading and literary exploration enhance your retirement years. Happy reading and discussing!

Courses and Workshops - Participating in Cultural Lessons and Events to Acquire New Skills

Retirement is an ideal time to pursue lifelong learning and acquire new skills. Courses and workshops offer retirees a wonderful opportunity to engage in cultural lessons and events that cater to their interests and passions. In this subsection, we explore the joys of enrolling in courses and workshops, where retirees can embrace continuous learning, delve into new subjects, and embark on exciting educational adventures.

Lifelong Learning and Personal Growth: Participating in courses and workshops promotes lifelong learning, fostering a sense of intellectual curiosity and personal growth during retirement. Whether it's learning a new language, mastering a musical instrument, or exploring art history, each new skill acquired enriches the retiree's life and broadens their horizons.

Cultural Immersion and Appreciation: Courses and workshops centered around cultural topics allow retirees to immerse themselves in the traditions, customs, and artistic expressions of different cultures. From dance lessons inspired by diverse world cultures to cooking classes that celebrate international cuisines, cultural courses offer an opportunity to appreciate the beauty and diversity of human heritage.

Acquiring Practical Skills: Beyond cultural topics, courses and workshops also provide opportunities to acquire practical skills that are useful in everyday life. From computer classes that improve digital literacy to gardening workshops that enhance green thumbs, retirees can develop skills that bring both enjoyment and practicality to their retirement lifestyle.

Connecting with Passionate Instructors: Enrolling in courses and workshops often means learning from passionate and knowledgeable instructors. These experts provide valuable guidance and inspiration, creating a supportive learning environment that encourages retirees to explore their interests and excel in their chosen pursuits.

Social Engagement and Community: Participating in courses and workshops fosters social engagement and creates a sense of community. Sharing the learning journey with like-minded individuals provides opportunities for networking, making new friends, and building meaningful connections. Whether in-person or virtual, the shared educational experience enhances the joy of learning.

Flexibility and Adapting to Interests: Courses and workshops offer flexibility in scheduling and subject matter, allowing retirees to tailor their learning experiences to align with their interests and preferences. Whether exploring a new hobby, honing existing talents, or diving into academic subjects of curiosity, retirees can customize their learning journey to suit their individual goals.

Conclusion

Courses and workshops open the door to continuous learning and skill acquisition during retirement. Embracing cultural lessons and educational events enriches the retiree's life by nurturing their intellectual curiosity and appreciation for diverse topics. Engaging in these educational adventures not only expands knowledge but also brings joy, inspiration, and a sense of personal achievement. So, enroll in a course, sign up for a workshop, and let the joy of learning lead you to new discoveries and meaningful experiences during your retirement years. Happy learning and growing!

CHAPTER 9: SOCIALIZATION AND COMMUNITY

Friend Meetups - Organizing Dinners, Parties, and Social Gatherings to Nurture Friendships

Socialization and community engagement play a vital role in enriching retirement life. Friend meetups offer retirees the opportunity to nurture existing friendships and forge new connections in a warm and convivial setting. This subsection explores the joys of organizing dinners, parties, and social gatherings, where retirees can come together to celebrate each other's company and create cherished memories.

Celebrating Togetherness: Friend meetups provide a delightful occasion to celebrate togetherness and the bond of friendship. Whether organizing intimate dinners at home, hosting lively parties, or planning casual get-togethers, these gatherings create an atmosphere of joy, camaraderie, and shared experiences.

Fostering Lasting Friendships: Retirement is an excellent time to invest in meaningful friendships that stand the test of time. Friend meetups offer a nurturing space to strengthen bonds and develop deeper connections with friends who share similar interests and values.

Creating Lasting Memories: The memories created during friend meetups become precious treasures that retirees can cherish for years to come. From laughter-filled evenings to heartwarming conversations, each gathering leaves a lasting imprint of joy and camaraderie.

Exploring New Activities Together: Friend meetups are an opportunity to explore new activities and hobbies together. Whether attending cultural events, embarking on group outings, or trying out a shared interest, engaging in these experiences deepens the bond between friends and creates unique and unforgettable moments.

Supporting Each Other Through Life's Journey: During retirement, friend meetups become a pillar of support through life's ups and downs. As retirees navigate new challenges and experiences, having a strong network of friends provides emotional support, empathy, and understanding.

Embracing Diversity and Inclusivity: Friend meetups often encompass a diverse group of friends from different backgrounds and life experiences. Embracing this diversity fosters inclusivity and broadens perspectives, creating a dynamic and supportive social circle.

Conclusion

Friend meetups are a cornerstone of socialization and community engagement during retirement. Organizing dinners, parties, and social gatherings allows retirees to nurture friendships, celebrate togetherness, and create lasting memories. As retirees come together to share laughter, experiences, and support, these gatherings become a source of joy and enrichment in their retirement journey. So, reach out to friends, plan those gatherings, and let the spirit of friendship and camaraderie light up your retirement years. Here's to many more cherished friend meetups and the lifelong bonds they create. Cheers to friendship and community!

Interest Groups - Joining Hobby or Activity Clubs to Meet Like-Minded Individuals

Retirement offers the perfect opportunity to explore and indulge in hobbies and activities that bring joy and fulfillment. Interest groups provide retirees with a wonderful way to connect with like-minded individuals who share common passions and pursuits. This subsection explores the joys of joining hobby or activity clubs, where retirees can foster new friendships, share experiences, and engage in meaningful activities together.

Discovering Shared Passions: Interest groups bring together individuals who have a genuine interest in a specific hobby or activity. Whether it's gardening, photography, hiking, painting, playing musical instruments, or any other shared pursuit, retirees can find a club that resonates with their passions, providing a platform for exploring and deepening their interests.

Nurturing Camaraderie: Joining an interest group creates an instant sense of camaraderie among members. Shared passions form the basis for conversations, and the common enthusiasm for the hobby fosters a warm and welcoming environment. This camaraderie enhances the social aspect of retirement and contributes to a sense of belonging within the group.

Regular Social Engagement: Interest groups often schedule regular meetups, activities, or events, providing retirees with consistent opportunities for social engagement. Whether it's weekly meetings, monthly outings, or special events, these gatherings offer a structured and enjoyable way to stay socially active and connected.

Skill Enhancement and Learning: Participating in interest groups allows retirees to continually enhance their skills and knowledge in their chosen hobbies or activities. Learning from more experienced members or participating in workshops and demonstrations within the group can further deepen retirees' expertise and passion for their shared interests.

A Sense of Purpose: Being part of an interest group provides retirees with a sense of purpose and motivation. Engaging in activities they are passionate about brings joy and fulfillment to their daily lives, contributing to a positive and vibrant retirement experience.

Opportunities for Collaboration and Contribution: Interest groups may collaborate on projects or contribute to the community through their shared interests. Whether it's organizing events, volunteering, or showcasing their talents to others, the group's collective efforts can have a meaningful and positive impact.

Conclusion

Interest groups offer retirees a fulfilling and socially engaging way to pursue their passions and interests during retirement. By joining hobby or activity clubs, retirees can connect with like-minded individuals, nurture new friendships, and share their enthusiasm for the hobbies they love. Engaging in regular meetups and activities allows retirees to continuously learn, grow, and find a sense of belonging within their interest groups. So, seek out those clubs, explore your passions, and let the camaraderie and shared experiences of interest groups enrich your retirement journey. Here's to many enjoyable moments of friendship and discovery with your fellow hobby enthusiasts!

Mentoring and Volunteering - Sharing Experiences and Knowledge with Younger Generations

Retirement offers retirees the opportunity to give back to their communities and make a positive impact on younger generations. Mentoring and volunteering are fulfilling ways for retirees to share their wealth of experiences, skills, and knowledge with others. This subsection explores the joys of mentoring and volunteering, where retirees can become valuable mentors and contribute to the growth and development of the next generation.

Becoming Valuable Mentors: Retirees possess a lifetime of experiences and wisdom that can benefit younger individuals seeking guidance and support. Mentoring allows retirees to act as valuable mentors, offering insights and advice gained from navigating various stages of life and careers. Serving as mentors creates meaningful connections and fosters a sense of purpose in retirees' lives.

Passing Down Knowledge and Skills: Volunteering provides retirees with an opportunity to pass down their expertise and skills to younger generations. Whether it's teaching a craft, sharing professional knowledge, or providing guidance in academic subjects, retirees can contribute to the development of future leaders and professionals.

Making a Positive Impact: Mentoring and volunteering allow retirees to make a positive impact on the lives of others, leaving a lasting legacy of support and encouragement. The knowledge and guidance shared with younger generations can empower individuals to achieve their goals and reach their full potential.

Fostering Inter-Generational Connections: Mentoring and volunteering create bridges between generations, fostering inter-generational connections and understanding. These interactions bring diverse age groups together, promoting empathy, mutual respect, and a deeper appreciation for each other's perspectives.

Contributing to Community Growth: Through volunteering, retirees contribute to the growth and development of their communities. By sharing their time and expertise with local organizations, schools, or non-profit groups, retirees actively participate in initiatives that address community needs and foster positive change.

Personal Fulfillment and Well-Being: Engaging in mentoring and volunteering activities brings personal fulfillment and a sense of well-being to retirees. The act of giving back and helping others can boost self-esteem, reduce stress, and create a profound sense of purpose and fulfillment in retirement.

Conclusion

Mentoring and volunteering offer retirees a meaningful way to share their experiences, knowledge, and skills with younger generations, making a positive impact on the lives of others. By becoming mentors and volunteers, retirees contribute to community growth and foster inter-generational connections.

Engaging in these fulfilling activities not only benefits the recipients but also brings personal fulfillment, purpose, and joy to retirees' lives. So, embrace the role of mentor, embrace volunteer opportunities, and let your guidance and support empower the next generation. Here's to a future filled with growth, learning, and positive change, all inspired by your valuable contributions!

CHAPTER 10: MINDFUL WELLNESS AND MEDITATION

Mindfulness practices: Embracing mindfulness techniques for stress reduction and mental clarity

In the fast-paced world of retirement, it's easy to get caught up in the whirlwind of activities and forget to take a moment for yourself. This is where mindfulness practices come in, offering a pathway to inner peace and mental clarity. Mindfulness involves being fully present in the moment, acknowledging your thoughts and feelings without judgment. By embracing mindfulness techniques, you can reduce stress, enhance your well-being, and make the most of your retirement journey.

The Power of Mindful Breathing: One of the simplest yet most effective mindfulness practices is mindful breathing. Find a quiet space, sit comfortably, and focus your attention on your breath. Observe each inhalation and exhalation, noticing how your body responds to the rhythmic flow of air. If your mind starts to wander, gently bring your focus back to your breath. This practice not only calms the mind but also connects you to the present moment.

Mindful Walking and Movement: Combine the benefits of physical activity with mindfulness by practicing mindful walking or gentle exercises like Tai Chi and Qi Gong. During a mindful walk, pay attention to each step, the sensation of your feet touching the ground, and the environment around you. Similarly, Tai Chi and Qi Gong involve slow, deliberate movements that promote relaxation and balance, fostering a sense of calm and well-being.

Meditation for Inner Calm: Meditation is a powerful tool for cultivating inner calm and mental clarity. Find a quiet space, sit or lie down comfortably, and close your eyes. Focus on your breath, a mantra, or a specific object of meditation. As thoughts arise, acknowledge them without judgment and let them pass like clouds in the sky. Regular meditation practice can lead to reduced anxiety, improved focus, and an overall sense of inner peace.

Mindful Eating: Retirement is an excellent time to savor the joys of food and eating mindfully can enhance this experience. Engage your senses fully when eating by appreciating the colors, textures, and flavors of your meal. Chew slowly and savor each bite, being fully present with the nourishment it provides. Mindful eating not only enhances your dining experience but can also promote healthier eating habits.

Gratitude and Mindfulness: Practicing gratitude goes hand in hand with mindfulness. Take a moment each day to reflect on the things you are thankful for, whether it's the beauty of nature, cherished memories, or the presence of loved ones. Cultivating gratitude can shift your focus towards the positive aspects of life, promoting a sense of contentment and well-being.

Mindful Technology Use: While technology offers exciting opportunities for retirees, it's essential to use it mindfully. Limit screen time and avoid multitasking when engaging with digital devices. Instead, savor the experiences they offer, such as virtual travel experiences or online learning courses. Use technology as a tool for enrichment and creativity rather than a source of distraction.

Conclusion

Mindfulness practices can be a transformative addition to your retirement lifestyle, providing a deeper connection to the present moment and enhancing your overall well-being. Embrace the art of mindful breathing, meditation, and movement to find inner peace and reduce stress. Incorporate mindfulness into your everyday activities, whether it's eating, walking, or engaging with technology, to fully experience the joy and richness of your retirement journey. By embracing mindfulness, you'll be better equipped to savor each day's adventures and lead a fulfilling life during your golden years.

Tai Chi and Qi Gong: Exploring the Benefits of these Gentle, Meditative Movements for Balance and Relaxation

In the quest for mindful wellness during retirement, Tai Chi and Qi Gong stand out as two ancient practices that offer profound benefits for both body and mind. Rooted in Chinese tradition, these gentle, meditative movements have been cherished for centuries as powerful tools for achieving balance, relaxation, and overall well-being. Let's delve into the world of Tai Chi and Qi Gong to discover the transformative effects they can bring to your retirement years.

The Essence of Tai Chi and Qi Gong: Tai Chi and Qi Gong are ancient mind-body practices that emphasize slow, flowing movements, deep breathing, and mindfulness. While they have distinct origins, both share a common foundation in Traditional Chinese Medicine and Daoist philosophy. Tai Chi is often described as a martial art in slow motion, characterized by continuous, circular movements that help in cultivating strength, flexibility, and inner harmony. Qi Gong, on the other hand, focuses on the cultivation and balance of the body's vital life force, known as "Qi" or "Chi," through specific postures, breathwork, and mental focus.

Balance and Flexibility: One of the key benefits of Tai Chi and Qi Gong is their ability to improve balance and flexibility. As we age, maintaining balance becomes crucial in preventing falls and maintaining mobility. The deliberate, controlled movements in

Tai Chi and Qi Gong help strengthen the muscles responsible for balance while enhancing proprioception—the awareness of one's body in space. Over time, practitioners often experience increased stability and a reduced risk of falls.

Stress Reduction and Relaxation: Retirement can sometimes bring its own set of stressors, and Tai Chi and Qi Gong can serve as invaluable tools for relaxation and stress reduction. The slow, intentional movements accompanied by deep, rhythmic breathing induce a state of calmness and mindfulness. As you flow through the movements, you may find that worries and tension melt away, leaving you with a profound sense of tranquility.

Enhancing Mindfulness and Mental Clarity: Both Tai Chi and Qi Gong demand focused attention and mental presence. By shifting your focus to the movements, breath, and sensations within your body, you enter a state of heightened mindfulness. Practicing mindfulness regularly can lead to improved cognitive function, enhanced clarity of thought, and a greater ability to remain centered in the face of life's challenges.

Low-Impact Exercise for All Fitness Levels: One of the beauties of Tai Chi and Qi Gong is that they are low-impact practices suitable for individuals of all ages and fitness levels. Whether you're an active retiree or new to physical exercise, these practices can be adapted to your abilities and needs. They offer a gentle, nurturing form of exercise that can be enjoyed by seniors seeking to stay active and healthy without putting strain on joints and muscles.

Cultivating Mind-Body Connection: Tai Chi and Qi Gong encourage a deep connection between the mind and body. As you engage in the graceful movements and synchronize them with your breath, you become more attuned to the signals your body sends. This heightened awareness can lead to a better understanding of your body's needs and an increased sense of self-awareness.

Conclusion

Tai Chi and Qi Gong are beautiful and accessible paths to mindful wellness during retirement. By embracing these ancient practices, you can experience improved balance, enhanced flexibility, reduced stress, and a profound sense of relaxation. As you flow through the meditative movements, you'll discover the deep connection between your mind and body, fostering a harmonious and balanced existence. Whether you practice individually or join a group, Tai Chi and Qi Gong can be transformative companions on your journey towards a fulfilling and enriching retirement lifestyle.

Wellness retreats: Discovering rejuvenating retreats to nourish the mind, body, and spirit

Retirement offers a precious opportunity to focus on self-care and overall well-being. One of the most rewarding ways to achieve this is by embarking on a wellness retreat—a sanctuary of serenity and rejuvenation. Wellness retreats are immersive experiences designed to nourish the mind, body, and spirit, providing a holistic approach to health and self-discovery. Let's explore the enchanting world of wellness retreats and how they can enrich your retirement journey.

The Essence of Wellness Retreats: Wellness retreats are carefully curated programs set in idyllic locations, such as serene nature reserves, beachfront resorts, or tranquil mountain retreats. These retreats offer a perfect blend of activities that promote physical health, mental clarity, and emotional balance. From yoga and meditation sessions to wholesome gourmet meals and holistic therapies, each element is thoughtfully designed to support your well-being and personal growth.

Mindfulness and Stress Relief: At the core of many wellness retreats lies the practice of mindfulness and stress relief. Engaging in guided meditation sessions or mindfulness workshops can help you reconnect with the present moment, leaving behind the worries and pressures of everyday life. The tranquil environment of a wellness retreat creates an ideal setting for you to find inner peace, recharge, and realign your priorities.

Physical Wellness and Fitness: Wellness retreats offer a plethora of physical activities tailored to all fitness levels. You can participate in rejuvenating yoga classes to enhance flexibility and strength or engage in invigorating hikes to connect with nature. Some retreats even offer dance classes, aqua aerobics, or outdoor workouts, ensuring you have opportunities to move your body and stay active during your retreat experience.

Spa Therapies and Relaxation: Indulge in luxurious spa therapies and relaxation sessions that pamper your body and soothe your senses. Wellness retreats often include massages, facials, and body treatments to promote relaxation and alleviate tension. These therapies not only rejuvenate your physical body but also contribute to an overall sense of well-being.

Nourishing Cuisine: At wellness retreats, you'll be treated to nourishing and delectable cuisine that supports your health goals. Wholesome, locally sourced ingredients are often used to create meals that are both nutritious and flavorful. From plant-based dishes to balanced gourmet feasts, you'll embark on a culinary journey that complements your desire for holistic wellness.

Opportunities for Self-Reflection and Growth: Retirement is an ideal time for self-reflection and personal growth, and wellness retreats provide the ideal environment for this inner exploration. Through workshops, group discussions, and private contemplation, you can gain insights into your life's purpose, set intentions for the future, and cultivate a deeper sense of self-awareness.

Conclusion

SERENA MITCHELL

Wellness retreats offer a magical escape from the routine and provide a transformative experience for retirees seeking to enhance their overall well-being. Immerse yourself in the serene ambiance of these retreats as you embrace mindfulness, engage in physical activities, and savor nourishing cuisine. Allow the gentle touch of spa therapies and the tranquility of meditation to revitalize your mind, body, and spirit. With each moment spent at a wellness retreat, you'll rediscover the essence of relaxation, self-discovery, and rejuvenation, creating cherished memories that will stay with you long after you return to your everyday life.

CHAPTER 11: TECHNOLOGY
AND DIGITAL ADVENTURES

Virtual travel experiences: Exploring the world from the comfort of home through virtual tours and experiences

In the digital age, retirement opens new avenues for exploration and adventure, even from the comfort of your own home. Virtual travel experiences have revolutionized the way we can connect with the world, offering an immersive journey to far-off places without leaving the living room. Through the magic of technology, you can embark on exciting virtual tours and experiences that satisfy your wanderlust and curiosity. Let's dive into the world of virtual travel and discover the wonders that await you on your digital adventures.

The Beauty of Virtual Tours: Virtual tours provide an authentic and interactive way to explore iconic landmarks, historic sites, and natural wonders. With just a few clicks, you can find yourself standing in front of the Eiffel Tower in Paris, strolling through the ancient ruins of Machu Picchu, or diving into the depths of the Great Barrier Reef. High-quality 360-degree imagery and informative audio guides make these virtual excursions almost as good as being there in person.

Cultural Immersion and Museums: Delve into the heart of culture and art through virtual visits to renowned museums and galleries worldwide. Wander through the Louvre in Paris to admire masterpieces like the Mona Lisa or explore the halls of the Metropolitan Museum of Art in New York City. Many museums offer virtual exhibitions that showcase diverse art collections, preserving cultural heritage for all to enjoy.

Unraveling Natural Wonders: Virtual travel takes you on a breathtaking journey to discover the Earth's most awe-inspiring natural wonders. From the majestic landscapes of the Grand Canyon to the mystical beauty of the Northern Lights in Iceland, you can witness the marvels of nature from any corner of the globe. Virtual travel provides a unique perspective on the world's most remarkable environments, fostering a deeper appreciation for our planet's diversity.

Historical Adventures and Architectural Marvels: History enthusiasts can indulge in virtual tours that unravel the secrets of ancient civilizations and architectural wonders. Walk the cobbled streets of Rome's Colosseum, wander through the mystique of Egypt's pyramids, or marvel at the grandeur of India's Taj Mahal. Virtual travel transcends time and space, allowing you to relive history's defining moments and architectural achievements.

Exploring Off-the-Beaten-Path Destinations: Venture off the beaten path with virtual travel experiences that introduce you to lesser-known gems. Explore charming villages, serene landscapes, and cultural enclaves that might not be on the typical tourist trail. Virtual travel's vast scope presents opportunities to uncover hidden treasures and connect with local communities from every corner of the globe.

Connecting with Others: Virtual travel isn't just a solo experience. Gather with friends and family online to embark on joint virtual adventures. Share experiences, discoveries, and emotions as you journey together through virtual landscapes. These shared moments can strengthen bonds and create lasting memories, even when you're physically apart.

Conclusion

Technology has opened a gateway to a world of digital adventures, providing retirees with a myriad of opportunities to explore and connect. Virtual travel experiences allow you to transcend physical limitations and immerse yourself in the wonders of our planet. Through virtual tours and experiences, you can fulfill your wanderlust, uncover cultural treasures, and appreciate the beauty of the natural world—all from the comfort of home. Embrace the digital age and let technology be your guide as you embark on captivating journeys that will leave you inspired and enriched during your retirement years.

Online Learning: Enrolling in Interactive Courses and Webinars to Acquire New Skills and Knowledge

Retirement marks a wonderful time to engage in lifelong learning and expand your horizons. With the advent of online learning platforms and webinars, acquiring new skills and knowledge has never been more accessible. Embracing the world of online education empowers retirees to explore diverse subjects, cultivate talents, and stay intellectually active. Let's delve into the realm of online learning and discover how it can invigorate your retirement journey.

A World of Learning at Your Fingertips: Online learning offers an extensive array of courses and webinars covering virtually every topic imaginable. From languages, arts, and sciences to hobbies, technology, and history, you can explore subjects that resonate with your passions and interests. Embrace the freedom to choose the courses that pique your curiosity and embark on a learning adventure that aligns with your individual goals.

Interactive and Engaging Courses: Online courses often feature interactive elements such as quizzes, discussions, and assignments that facilitate active learning. Engaging with course materials in this manner fosters a deeper understanding of the subject matter and enhances the overall learning experience. Many courses also provide opportunities to connect with instructors and fellow learners, fostering a sense of community and camaraderie in the digital classroom.

Flexible Learning at Your Own Pace: One of the greatest advantages of online learning is its flexibility. As a retiree, you have the freedom to structure your learning around your lifestyle and preferences. Whether you prefer to dive into a course intensively or take it slowly over time, online learning accommodates your schedule and pace. This flexibility allows you to strike the perfect balance between acquiring new knowledge and enjoying your retirement pursuits.

Nurturing Curiosity and Personal Growth: Lifelong learning nurtures curiosity and keeps your mind sharp and agile. Embracing new subjects and acquiring fresh skills can boost self-confidence and promote personal growth during your retirement years. Engaging in continuous learning not only enriches your intellectual life but also opens doors to new opportunities and activities.

Pursuing Hobbies and Creative Passions: Online learning platforms offer a treasure trove of courses dedicated to hobbies and creative pursuits. Whether you want to learn to play a musical instrument, improve your photography skills, or delve into the world of creative writing, there's an online course waiting for you. Embracing hobbies and creative passions can bring immense joy and fulfillment to your retirement journey.

Embracing Technology and Digital Literacy: Participating in online courses and webinars also presents an opportunity to enhance your digital literacy. As you navigate through virtual classrooms and interactive platforms, you'll become more comfortable with technology and its myriad applications. Strengthening your digital skills can enrich your retirement experience and open doors to further technological exploration.

Conclusion

Online learning is a powerful tool for retirees seeking to expand their knowledge, cultivate talents, and engage in lifelong learning. With a vast range of interactive courses and webinars at your disposal, you can explore diverse subjects, connect with like-minded individuals, and nurture your intellectual curiosity. Embrace the flexibility of online learning to fit your lifestyle and pace, and revel in the joy of acquiring new skills and knowledge during your retirement journey. As you embark on this enriching digital adventure, you'll discover that the pursuit of knowledge knows no bounds, and the world of learning remains forever at your fingertips.

Digital Creativity: Embracing Technology to Express Artistic Talents through Digital Art, Music, and Storytelling

Retirement is the perfect time to unleash your inner artist and explore new avenues of creative expression. With the rise of technology, digital creativity has become an accessible and exciting realm for retirees to dive into. Embracing digital tools allows you to tap into your artistic talents and breathe life into your imagination through digital art, music, and storytelling. Let's venture into the world of digital creativity and discover the limitless possibilities it offers for self-expression and artistic fulfillment.

Digital Art, Painting Without Boundaries: Digital art provides a canvas without constraints, offering endless possibilities for creative exploration. With drawing tablets, digital brushes, and powerful software, you can paint, sketch, and illustrate with remarkable precision. Whether you're a seasoned artist or just beginning your artistic journey, digital tools empower you to experiment with colors, textures, and styles in ways that traditional media may not allow.

Music Composition in the Digital Realm: Technology has revolutionized music creation, enabling aspiring musicians and composers to bring their melodies to life. Digital audio workstations (DAWs) offer a plethora of virtual instruments and effects, allowing you to compose, arrange, and produce music with ease. Whether you dream of composing symphonies, crafting electronic beats, or simply recording your own melodies, digital music production unleashes the maestro within you.

Digital Storytelling: From Words to Multimedia: In the digital age, storytelling transcends traditional written narratives. Digital storytelling embraces multimedia elements such as images, videos, and animations to captivate audiences and convey emotions. You can craft interactive digital stories or explore the world of e-books and digital publishing to share your tales with the world. Digital storytelling empowers you to share your experiences, imagination, and wisdom in compelling and innovative ways.

Exploring Graphic Design and Visual Communication: Delve into the realm of graphic design and visual communication using digital tools. Create stunning graphics for social media, design personalized greeting cards, or develop captivating visual presentations. Digital design software empowers you to transform ideas into visually striking creations, allowing you to communicate messages and stories through images and graphics.

Collaborative Artistic Projects: The digital world fosters collaboration and connection with like-minded individuals. Join online artistic communities or participate in collaborative projects that unite artists from diverse backgrounds. Engaging with others in the digital realm not only fuels your creativity but also exposes you to different perspectives and techniques, enriching your own artistic journey.

Preserving and Sharing Creative Works: Digital creativity offers the advantage of easy preservation and sharing of your artistic endeavors. With digital files and cloud storage, your creations can be safely stored and easily accessed at any time. Share your digital art, music, and storytelling with friends, family, and the world, embracing the joy of sharing your creativity and leaving a lasting artistic legacy.

Conclusion

Digital creativity has opened a universe of possibilities for retirees seeking to express their artistic talents and nurture their creativity. Whether you immerse yourself in digital art, compose music, or craft multimedia storytelling, technology empowers you to explore and create without boundaries. Embrace the digital tools and platforms that resonate with your artistic vision and let your imagination soar in the boundless world of digital creativity. With every stroke of the digital brush, every musical note composed, and every story told, you'll discover the profound fulfillment that comes from expressing yourself and leaving a unique artistic mark on the digital canvas of the world.

CONCLUSION

"Fun Things to Do in Retirement: 365 Daily Discoveries of Exciting Adventures and Healthy Pursuits for the Young-at-Heart Seniors" has taken you on a journey of exploration, adventure, and self-discovery. From embarking on exciting new challenges to nurturing your creative passions, this comprehensive guide has shown that retirement is far from a time of idleness—it's a canvas brimming with endless opportunities for growth and fulfillment.

As you embrace the essence of adventure in Chapter 1, venturing into new horizons and planning your calendar of activities, you'll find that retirement is the perfect time to immerse yourself in exciting pursuits that ignite your spirit.

The chapters on nature adventures, creative and artistic pursuits, fitness and wellness, travel and global adventures, cooking and gastronomy, DIY projects and crafts, cultural experiences, socialization and community, and mindful wellness and meditation have unveiled an abundance of activities to engage your body, mind, and soul. Whether you choose to hike through scenic trails, unleash your inner artist, travel to new destinations, or participate in social gatherings, each experience adds color to the tapestry of your retirement life.

Furthermore, technology and digital adventures invite you to explore a world of virtual travel, online learning, and digital creativity, proving that age is no barrier to embracing technology for enrichment and exploration.

In the culmination of your retirement journey, you'll come to appreciate that life's adventures never cease, and retirement becomes an invitation to embrace every moment with vitality, joy, and a pursuit of personal growth. With each chapter offering a diverse range of activities, you're encouraged to curate a life that reflects your passions and dreams.

As you venture into the world of "Fun Things to Do in Retirement: 365 Daily Discoveries of Exciting Adventures and Healthy Pursuits for the Young-at-Heart Seniors", seize the opportunities, embrace the challenges, and immerse yourself in the joy of discovering the best version of yourself during your golden years. Whether you're exploring new horizons, cultivating mindfulness, pursuing creative endeavors, or connecting with communities, this book empowers you to craft a retirement lifestyle that is uniquely yours.

So, as you close this book, take with you the belief that retirement is not a destination; it's a magnificent journey where every day holds the promise of adventure, joy, and boundless possibilities. Embrace the spirit of "365 Fun Things to Do in Retirement," and let the next chapter of your life be filled with fulfillment, excitement, and the pursuit of happiness. Remember, life's adventures are forever at your fingertips—go forth and make the most of each day's journey!

Printed in Great Britain
by Amazon